Depression in New Mothers, Volume 1

Depression in New Mothers, Volume 1: Causes, Consequences, and Risk Factors provides a comprehensive, evidence-based approach to understanding symptoms and risk factors of depression, anxiety, and posttraumatic stress disorder (PTSD) in perinatal women, which are common complications of childbirth.

To effectively intervene, health professionals must be aware of these conditions and ready to identify them in mothers they see. Written by a psychologist and International Board–Certified Lactation Consultant, this fourth edition is expanded into two complementary volumes: the first focuses on causes and consequences of poor perinatal mental health, and the second, on screening and treatment. This volume integrates recent research on:

- Feeding methods and sleep location for mother–infant sleep
- Traumatic birth experiences
- Infant temperament, illness, and prematurity
- Violence, discrimination, and adversity
- The dysphoric milk-ejection reflex (D-MER)
- COVID-19, military sexual trauma, immigration/refugee status, and the impact of war, displacement, and terrorist attacks

Depression in New Mothers, Volume 1 includes mothers' stories throughout, which provide examples of principles described in studies. Each chapter highlights key research findings and clinical takeaways. It is an essential resource for all healthcare practitioners working with mothers in the perinatal period, including nurses, midwives, doctors, lactation consultants, and psychologists.

Kathleen A. Kendall-Tackett is a health psychologist and International Board–Certified Lactation Consultant. Dr. Kendall-Tackett is the Editor-in-Chief of the journal *Psychological Trauma*. She is a Fellow of the American Psychological Association in Health and Trauma Psychology, the Past President of the APA Division of Trauma Psychology and is a member of Postpartum Support International's President's Advisory Committee. Dr. Kendall-Tackett specializes in women's health research, including breastfeeding, depression, trauma, and health psychology. This is her 41st book.

Depression in New Mothers, Volume 1

Causes, Consequences, and Risk Factors

Fourth Edition

Kathleen A. Kendall-Tackett

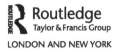
Routledge
Taylor & Francis Group

LONDON AND NEW YORK

Designed cover image: Getty Images

Fourth edition published 2024
by Routledge
4 Park Square, Milton Park, Abingdon, Oxon, OX14 4RN

and by Routledge
605 Third Avenue, New York, NY 10158

Routledge is an imprint of the Taylor & Francis Group, an informa business

First edition published by Routledge 2005
Third edition published by Routledge 2016

British Library Cataloguing-in-Publication Data
A catalogue record for this book is available from the British Library

Library of Congress Cataloging-in-Publication Data
Names: Kendall-Tackett, Kathleen A., author.
Title: Depression in new mothers / Kathleen A. Kendall-Tackett.
Description: Fourth edition. | Milton Park, Abingdon, Oxon ; New York, NY :
    Routledge, 2024. | Includes bibliographical references and index.
Contents: Volume 1. Causes, consequences, and risk factors —
Identifiers: LCCN 2023024798 | ISBN 9781032532776 (volume 1 ; hardback) |
    ISBN 9781032532752 (volume 1 ; paperback) |
    ISBN 9781003411246 (volume 1 ; ebook)
Subjects: LCSH: Postpartum depression.
Classification: LCC RG852 .K448 2024 | DDC 618.7/6—dc23/eng/20230717
LC record available at https://lccn.loc.gov/2023024798

ISBN: 978-1-032-53277-6 (hbk)
ISBN: 978-1-032-53275-2 (pbk)
ISBN: 978-1-003-41124-6 (ebk)

DOI: 10.4324/9781003411246

Typeset in Sabon
by Apex CoVantage, LLC

Contents

Author Biography

Dr. Kendall-Tackett is a health psychologist and International Board-Certified Lactation Consultant and the CEO of Praeclarus Press, a small press specializing in women's health. Dr. Kendall-Tackett is the editor-in-chief of the journal *Psychological Trauma* and was the Founding Editor-in-Chief of *Clinical Lactation*. She is Fellow of the American Psychological Association in Health and Trauma Psychology, is Past President of the APA Division of Trauma Psychology, and is on APA's Publications and Communications Board.

Dr. Kendall-Tackett specializes in women's health research, including breastfeeding, depression, trauma, and health psychology, and has won many awards for her work, including the 2019 President's Award for Outstanding Contributions to the Field of Trauma Psychology from the American Psychological Association. Dr. Kendall-Tackett has authored more than 490 articles or chapters and is the author or editor of 41 books. Her most recent books include *Breastfeeding Doesn't Need to Suck* (2022, American Psychological Association), *Women's Mental Health Across the Lifespan* (2017, Routledge US, with Lesia Ruglass), and *The Phantom of the Opera: A Social History of the World's Most Popular Musical* (2018, Praeclarus). This is her 41st book.

Kathleen A. Kendall-Tackett, PhD, IBCLC, FAPA

Foreword

In this revised version of *Depression in New Mothers* written by Kathleen A. Kendall Tackett, almost 80% of the content is new. Since each chapter contains an abstract, an introduction, key findings, and take-home messages, in addition to summaries of articles, the reader can easily get to the core of the information presented in the chapters. Therefore, everybody interested in postpartum depression and maternal psychological health should read this valuable book.

The structure of the book is logical. It starts with a description of the objective and subjective signs of depression after birth. Maternal depression occurs all over the world, although the frequency of the condition differs between countries. Adverse outcomes for mothers (and sometimes fathers) and their newborns caused by postpartum depression are also described.

Several chapters summarize risk factors for maternal depression. There are most certainly individual predispositions. Psychiatric history, exposure to previous trauma (ranging from sexual abuse to birth trauma), as well premature birth and the newborn's temperament may all contribute to maternal depression. Also, a plethora of different complex environmental and socioeconomical factors facilitates the occurrence of maternal depression.

Kathleen A. Kendall-Tackett also notes that premature labor increased during the corona epidemic in the US, which is one of the factors that may coincide with maternal depression. In Scandinavia, it was the reverse. The frequency of premature birth decreased during COVID. Why? Perhaps because the frequency of women working full-time differs between the US and Scandinavia. In the US, the stress of isolation at home had a negative impact on mothers and was associated with more premature births and depression. In Scandinavia, it was protective to stay at home, maybe because leaving home and going to the working place, at some level, is stressful during pregnancy. These different associations highlight the complex relationships between internal and external factors that are associated with maternal depression.

The book also describes factors that may reduce the risk of maternal depression, including the preventive role that mother's own oxytocin may play. Breastfeeding, exclusive breastfeeding in particular, is labelled nature's own medicine for postpartum maternal depression, as it is linked to a lower frequency of depression. Social support is also healing, however, only if the "support" is experienced as positive and accepted by the mother. Interestingly, both breastfeeding and positive relationships/social support are linked to a release of oxytocin in the mother's brain, which alleviates fear and pain, as well as stress and inflammation, which promote depression. Therefore, breastfeeding and social support will, via a release of the mother's own oxytocin, decrease the risk of developing maternal depression. Note that administration of synthetic oxytocin as a nasal spray does not prevent maternal postpartum depression.

Kathleen A. Kendall-Tackett is a psychologist who has devoted a large part of her life to studying and writing about breastfeeding, and she is also an International Board-Certified Lactation Consultant (IBCLC). She understands the complex situation of motherhood and is the absolute expert on women's mental health in the postpartum period, including consequences of previous traumatic experiences. She also understands the protective role of oxytocin via breastfeeding and social support. Kathy Kendall-Tackett is not only very knowledgeable but also has a fabulous verbal talent and knows, like nobody else, how to explain even complex relationships in engaging, simple terms.

Read this book and you will know everything there is about maternal depression!

Kerstin Uvnäs Moberg

MD, PhD, Professor of Physiology

Preface

Depression in new mothers is a common complication of childbirth that isolates them when they most need help. Early motherhood is difficult, but mothers sometimes think it is easy for everyone else—and social media does not help. How can struggling mothers tell people the truth? So they suffer in silence.

Some argue that modern civilization changed our lives in ways that put new mothers at risk (Hahn-Holbrook & Haselton, 2014). Mothers in industrialized countries often wean early, are deficient in omega-3 fatty acids and vitamin D, exercise less, and isolate themselves from kin networks. There is a fundamental mismatch between modern civilization and the way motherhood has been for millennia.

The unfortunate fact is that depression, anxiety, and posttraumatic stress disorder are common in pregnant and postpartum women, with some groups at especially high risk. Yet practitioners often act as if postpartum mental illness is rare. It is not.

It has been my tremendous honor to work on various editions of this book since 1992. I've had a front-row seat to the tremendous strides we have made. So much has changed since I wrote that first edition.[1] Thousands of new studies from around the world have described incidence of depression and the range of factors that increase mothers' risk. Groups at particularly high risk include immigrants and asylum seekers, women with abusive partners, women in the military, and ethnic/minority women. We have also lived through a pandemic that wreaked havoc on new mothers' mental health. Mothers have lived through hurricanes, earthquakes, terrorist attacks, and war. As a result, they have high rates of depression, anxiety, and posttraumatic stress disorder, but also tremendous resilience. Researchers have also looked beyond mothers and babies. New fathers can also be depressed, even if their partners are not. I have included these studies as well.

Stress vs Oxytocin

In the 2nd edition, I introduced inflammation as an underlying cause of perinatal depression. It is not simply a risk factor but *the* risk factor, the one that underlies all the others (Kendall-Tackett, 2007). In this edition, I include inflammation's counter-mechanism: oxytocin. To say it simply, if the oxytocin system is activated, inflammation is suppressed, which lowers the risk of depression. Conversely, if stress is activated, it suppresses oxytocin.

The oxytocin vs stress systems also explains why feeding method is relevant to mothers' mental health. Breastfeeding activates the oxytocin system, which lowers the risk for depression—if it is going well. If it is not, the stress system activates, suppressing oxytocin and increasing their risk for depression. Putting aside, for a moment, arguments about what to feed babies, my concern is, can we protect mothers? That is why feeding method needs to be part of the conversation about perinatal mental health. My best-case scenario is mental health practitioners and lactation consultants working together to support new mothers' mental health—and their breastfeeding goals.

I am particularly excited about this edition. There have been many real breakthroughs that help us understand the complexities of mental health in the perinatal period. The more we know, the better we are equipped to help.

Two Volumes for This Edition

For this edition, we split the book into two volumes. There is so much new research, and a single volume would have been impossibly long and way too much to read. This first volume focuses on depression risk factors and consequences but also describes comorbid conditions. The second volume focuses on assessment and treatment.

I have also made some structural changes to the text. I highlighted key findings and added clinical takeaways. The new research is amazing. I want to do all that I can to make it accessible. You can skim the key findings and then read about the studies in more detail. The clinical takeaways highlight how the information is relevant for practice.

You have before you an opportunity to make a real difference in the lives of mothers, babies, and whole families. When mental illness impacts one family member, it affects the entire unit. You can stop that downward progression.

The late pediatrician Dr. Ray Helfer once described the perinatal period as a "window of opportunity" in our work with young families. At no other time are they as interested and willing to learn. If you can identify postpartum depression, anxiety, or PTSD and help mothers get the treatment they need, they won't continue to suffer. It's a worthy goal. My goal is to equip you to do just that.

Kathleen A. Kendall-Tackett
Amarillo, Texas
February 2023

Note

1 Kendall-Tackett, K. A. *Postpartum depression: A comprehensive approach for nurses* (Sage Publications, 1993).

Section I

Symptoms, Incidence, and Consequences

1 Symptoms of Postpartum Depression and Comorbid Conditions

Depression is common in new mothers and happens to mothers worldwide. Most research continues to focus on depression, but many studies now include comorbid conditions, such as anxiety and posttraumatic stress disorder (PTSD). As I describe the studies in each section, I will include any co-occurring conditions. If studies focus primarily on anxiety or PTSD, I will include those as well. Where relevant, longitudinal studies that start during pregnancy and continue postpartum will also be included.

KEY FINDINGS

- New mothers' increased healthcare use can be a symptom of depression, anxiety, or PTSD.
- Depression and anxiety have high rates of co-occurrence, but some mothers have anxiety alone and would not be identified if practitioners only screened for depression.
- Obsessive thoughts about infant harm are not likely to lead to infant harm and differ from psychosis, which can lead to actual infant harm.
- Bipolar disorder is often the underlying condition in postpartum psychosis.

Postpartum Depression

Postpartum depression can manifest in a wide variety of symptoms, including sadness, anhedonia (the inability to experience pleasure), low self-esteem, and social withdrawal (American Psychiatric Association, 2022). Anxiety, anger, guilt, or mental fog can also be symptoms, as can pain, fatigue, sleep problems, and appetite disturbances. Symptoms can happen suddenly, as this mother describes.

> I just didn't feel like I had given birth. I felt disconnected from my body. I was up for 24 hours. I was crying hysterically. She wanted to eat a lot. I never was able to breastfeed. I was in the hospital crying. I didn't feel like her mother. I was very disconnected. I was freaking out. My friends kept telling me that it was the baby blues.

In a qualitative study of 12 women from Ghana, "thinking too much" was the predominant symptom of depression (Scorza et al., 2015).

> I don't sleep at night or in the day, because the eyes cannot close while the mind is still thinking.

DOI: 10.4324/9781003411246-2

You sleep small, and when those thoughts come into your mind, you cannot sleep anymore.

Their symptoms included body pain, trouble eating and sleeping, low milk supply, intrusive thoughts, social withdrawal, sadness, and tearfulness (Scorza et al., 2015). Fifty-eight percent believed that their condition would kill them or their babies, and 42% had suicidal thoughts. Like their Western counterparts, financial problems, family stress, lack of support, and problems with their partners all contributed to mothers' symptoms.

Increased Healthcare Use

Depression or anxiety increases the rate of healthcare use and can be a symptom (Williams & Koleva, 2018). For example, a study of 594 women in British Columbia found that women depressed at 4 weeks also describe their health as poor and were twice as likely to use healthcare often (Dennis, 2004). Similarly, a study of 591 low-income women in Bangladesh found that depression increased healthcare use and out-of-pocket expenses for health services (Hossain et al., 2020). Fifty-two percent were depressed. Depressed mothers sold possessions or borrowed money so they could access health services.

However, depressed mothers do not always seek healthcare. In a Canadian study of 665 mothers with infants 2 to 12 months old, depressed mothers did not use more healthcare services, including primary care, emergency department, or walk-in clinics (Anderson et al., 2008). Eleven percent had postpartum depressive symptoms, and 9% had postpartum anxiety.

Diagnostic Criteria for Major Depressive Disorder

While many mothers have depressive symptoms, to be diagnosed with major depressive disorder (MDD), they must meet criteria in the *Diagnostic and Statistical Manual-5 Text Revision* (DSM-5-TR) (American Psychiatric Association, 2022). Postpartum depression is not a distinct diagnosis, but clinicians can add "with postpartum onset" if it occurs in the first 4 weeks after birth. For major depression, women must have at least five of the following symptoms during the same 2-week period. The two most prominent symptoms are depressed mood and anhedonia (inability to experience pleasure). Other symptoms include significant weight loss or gain, changes in appetite, sleeping too much or too little, agitation or slowed motor activity, fatigue, feeling worthless or guilty, diminished concentration, indecisiveness, and frequent thoughts of death or suicide.

Symptoms must significantly impact their daily lives and should not be due to psychosis. Further, the woman's symptoms should not be due to physical illness; use of alcohol, medication, or illegal drugs; or normal bereavement, and she should never have had a manic or hypomanic episode. These symptoms can be by subjective report or others' observations and occur nearly every day (American Psychiatric Association, 2022).

Depression often co-occurs with other conditions, such as anxiety disorders, posttraumatic stress disorder, and possibly, bipolar disorder and psychosis (Cabizuca et al., 2009).

Postpartum Anxiety Disorders

Anxiety often co-occurs with depression but can occur alone. In fact, anxiety may be more common than depression. Postpartum anxiety disorders include panic disorders, generalized anxiety disorder, social phobia, and obsessive-compulsive disorder (Williams &

Koleva, 2018). PRAMS[1] data from Illinois and Maryland (*n* = 4,451) indicated that 18% of mothers had postpartum anxiety, and 35% of those mothers were also depressed (6% of the total) (Farr et al., 2014). Of the women who were depressed, 64% also had anxiety symptoms. Fifty-eight percent of women with depression and anxiety had three or more stressors. Twenty percent of women with anxiety had diabetes and women with diabetes were twice as likely to have anxiety as non-diabetic women.

A Canadian population survey (*n* = 6,558) found that 14% of women had anxiety symptoms and 18% had depressive symptoms (Gheorghe et al., 2021). If women had previously been depressed, they were 3.4 times more likely to have postpartum anxiety and 2.6 times more likely to have postpartum depression compared to women who had never been depressed. Women who rated their health as fair or poor were 2.4 times more likely to have anxiety and 2 times more likely to have depression compared to those who rated their health as excellent or very good.

A study from Croatia found that pregnancy was a high-risk time for anxiety, with or without comorbid depression (Rados et al., 2018). In their sample of 272 new mothers, 35% had anxiety during pregnancy, 17% had anxiety immediately postpartum, with 21% having anxiety at 6 weeks. Seventy-five percent of mothers with anxiety were also depressed. However, if mothers were only screened for depression, the 25% who only had anxiety would not have been identified.

A study from Japan included 99 pregnant women and assessed them during late pregnancy, and at 5 days and 12 months postpartum (Kokubu et al., 2012). Prenatal anxiety predicted postpartum depression and bonding failure, but depression during pregnancy did not. "Bonding failure" included positive responses to items such as "I resent my child" or "I feel nothing for my child," and negative responses to items such as "I feel loving towards my child" or "I enjoy doing things with my child."

Panic Disorder

Panic disorder is characterized by sudden, recurrent, and unpredictable panic attacks. Symptoms include palpitations, shortness of breath, chest pain, dizziness, fear of losing control, and fear of dying, and they tend to peak in minutes (Anda et al., 1999; Williams & Koleva, 2018). Mothers who have panic attacks use more healthcare, and panic disorder increases the risk of agoraphobia, where mothers are afraid to leave the house.

Panic disorder and depression also co-occur. In Ross and McLean's (2006) review, 50% of people with panic disorder also had major depression. A study from Australia of 1,507 pregnant women found that 9% reported intense anxiety or panic attacks, and 10% reported depressed mood between 6 and 9 months postpartum (Woolhouse et al., 2009). Mothers who had panic disorder and depression sought assistance more often than those with depression or anxiety alone.

Panic disorder was assessed retrospectively in 128 women from Germany, 93 of whom had had 195 pregnancies (Bandelow et al., 2006). Panic was more frequent postpartum than during pregnancy. Three percent of mothers reported that panic attacks decreased during their pregnancies, but 18% reported that they increased.

Obsessive-Compulsive Disorder

Obsessive-compulsive disorder (OCD) is characterized by recurrent, unwelcome thoughts, ideas, or doubts that give rise to anxiety and distress (obsessions). These thoughts often focus on accidentally harming their infants, and mothers feel guilt or shame for thinking these thoughts (Williams & Koleva, 2018). These obsessions lead to compulsions, which are excessive behavioral or mental acts to keep everyone safe (Abramowitz et al., 2003; Ross & McLean, 2006). Although data are limited, the postpartum prevalence of OCD is approximately 3% to 4% (Ross & McLean, 2006), but as many as 91% of new mothers have intrusive thoughts about their babies. Obsessions and depression co-occur about 50% of the time (Williams & Koleva, 2018). A population study of 763 English-speaking pregnant women assessed OCD during pregnancy and postpartum (Fairbrother et al., 2021). Nine percent had OCD at both 8 weeks and 6 months, which is higher than previous estimates in non-clinical samples.

In a sample of women with perinatal mood disorders ($n = 60$), 87% had obsessive thoughts and compulsive behaviors (Abramowitz et al., 2010). Most had mild symptoms, but 38% had clinically significant OCD, which was associated with both depression and anxiety. Women with higher depressive symptoms had significantly more obsessive-compulsive symptoms.

A prospective cohort study of 461 postpartum women from the 1990s found that 11% screened positive for OCD, while another 38% had subclinical obsessions and compulsions (Miller et al., 1993). Subclinical OCD was associated with both depression (24%) and state-trait anxiety (8%). The obsessions included fear of doing something embarrassing, harming others because they were not careful enough, being responsible for something terrible happening, dirt and germs, not saying just the right thing, losing things, being obsessive about symmetry or exactness, and feeling like they need to know or remember certain things. The compulsions included being bothered by certain sounds, noise, or mental images, having superstitious fears, washing hands excessively or in a ritualized way, checking that they did not make a mistake, and needing to re-read or rewrite things. The authors noted that nearly half of the women in their sample experienced postpartum obsessions and compulsions.

Obsessions about Infant Harm

In postpartum women, obsessive thoughts often focus on infant harm (Williams & Koleva, 2018). In a systematic review, obsession about accidentally harming their babies were common, including checking compulsions, self-reassurance, and seeking reassurance from others (Starcevic et al., 2020). This mother describes how she developed symptoms of OCD and panic disorder after a previous stillbirth and high-risk pregnancy. Her symptoms started 6 months postpartum.

> I was nervous about everything. About germs, development, baby care, all of it. I started having these thoughts about Zeke's safety. The scariest part were these weird thoughts about harming him myself. I was afraid to say anything to anybody. They terrified me. I kept hoping it would go away. It didn't. . . .
>
> My husband had an Employee Assistance Program that was also available to spouses. I didn't know where else to go, but I called them the next day when nobody else was there. I used a quiet voice and felt huge shame. . . . They got me set up with a counselor in my area who diagnosed me with postpartum depression. . . .
>
> That next counselor was a godsend. She talked to me about my expectations, reassured me that I wouldn't actually hurt my baby, and helped me know when it was time for antidepressants. I slowly got better.

I have since discovered, after several counselors, that I actually had postpartum OCD that was left untreated for far too long. I have experienced differing severity of OCD with every child since then (I now have 7 living children).

Even when there is depression but no OCD, approximately 40% of mothers report having obsessive thoughts (Ross & McLean, 2006). Some concern fears of hurting the baby with knives, or throwing the baby downstairs or out a window (Abramowitz et al., 2003). Other types of obsessive thoughts concern their babies dying in their sleep, or that they would sexually abuse or physically misplace them. Not surprisingly, obsessive thoughts can be very troubling to mothers, as this mother describes.

My postpartum depression was basically weird thoughts toward the baby, and he was a wonderful baby. The perfect baby. One time I had him on the bathroom floor with me. All of the sudden, I had this thought to kick the baby. This was the first weird thought I had toward him. My pediatrician told me that this was very normal. "You had a traumatic delivery." . . . I would have weird thoughts when I was breastfeeding. I was constantly worried that the baby would hit his head on the table. I was also scared to walk through the doorway, that he would hit his head. These thoughts would become obsessive. I was afraid if I told anyone, they'd take the baby away. I finally told my mom. She said it was normal and not to worry. This lasted around 5 months. . . . If I was ironing, I'd be terrified that the baby would be burned. Even if he was upstairs asleep in his bed. Then I would start to analyze my thoughts. "Am I thinking he'd be burned because I wanted him to be burned?" I was also scared of knives. . . . I didn't want to do these things. I couldn't understand why I was thinking this way. . . . These thoughts happened every day, all the time. Slowly, I had fewer thoughts. I'd think "there's no way he can hit his head when I'm holding him." . . . The hardest thing was I couldn't find anyone who had this experience. I knew about it, but I couldn't seem to find anyone who had been through it.

IS THERE A THREAT OF INFANT HARM?

Safety always must be a top concern, but if a mother has thoughts of infant harm, is she at risk for harming her baby? Speisman et al. (2011) distinguished obsessive thoughts of infant harm from psychosis, which can lead to actual infant harm. Psychotic symptoms are not present in OCD. In psychosis, thoughts of harm are consistent with a person's delusional thinking. A person acts out aggressive behavior because she believes she must do it (e.g., she believes her baby is possessed by the devil). In contrast, obsessive thoughts do not increase the risk of infant harm. These thoughts are unwanted and inconsistent with a person's normal behavior and are so distressing that people suffering from OCD will go to great lengths to keep these bad things from happening.

When speaking to a mother, say something like this: "It must be very distressing to you to have such thoughts. Many other women have these thoughts, and they do not mean that you are a bad mother or will harm your baby. These thoughts usually mean that you are experiencing severe stress, and it may help to talk with someone about it." Then you can offer some names of people who can help. This type of approach validates her experience while taking the problem seriously.

Unfortunately, there are times when you must take more drastic action. If you fear that the baby is in danger, you may be legally obligated to make a report to the department of social services or your local child protective agency. But in most cases, that will not be necessary.

Posttraumatic Stress Disorder

Posttraumatic stress disorder (PTSD) is another condition that often co-occurs with depression. Women may have pre-existing PTSD due to prior trauma, such as childhood adversities, sexual assault, partner violence, combat, or natural disaster. Birth can also cause it (see Chapter 10). Depression and PTSD share several diagnostic features, including diminished interest in significant activities, restricted range of affect, difficultly falling and staying asleep, difficulty with concentration, and restricted range of affect (Kendall-Tackett, 2014).

A review of 26 articles found that 3.3% of women have PTSD during pregnancy and 4% have postpartum PTSD (Cook et al., 2018). Postpartum PTSD was related to lower birthweight and lower rates of breastfeeding and can potentially influence the mother–infant relationship. A review of 78 studies found a wider range of postpartum PTSD, ranging from 3% in community samples to 16% in at-risk samples (Grekin & O'Hara, 2014). Postpartum PTSD was strongly related to depression. The history of trauma and infant complications were both risk factors. For racial/ethnic minority women, there was a stronger relationship between trauma and postpartum PTSD than there was for White women.

Even if women do not meet full criteria, they can still experience PTSD symptoms (American Psychiatric Association, 2022). PTSD will be described in more detail in Chapters 10 and 11, but what follows is a brief overview of its co-occurrence with postpartum depression (Cook et al., 2018). Seng and colleagues (Seng et al., 2009) found a 20% lifetime rate of PTSD in a sample of 1,581 pregnant women. Eight percent of the sample had current PTSD, but the rate for women on Medicaid was 14%. Women with PTSD were more likely to be African American teens with low education who were living in poverty and in high-crime neighborhoods. Eighty-six percent had violent partners, 85% had full or partial PTSD, and 12% had major depression. Childhood physical and sexual abuse were major risk factors for PTSD.

In this same sample, African American women had the highest rate of trauma exposure and PTSD ($n = 709$) (Seng, 2011). The rate of lifetime PTSD for African Americans was 24%, with current prevalence of 13% (compared to 3.5% for the predominantly White comparison group)—more than 4 times the rate than the comparison group.

PTSD Comorbid with Depression and Anxiety

Recent Canadian guidelines recommend screening all new mothers for posttraumatic stress disorder. (They already have mandatory screening for postpartum depression.) Sixty-five percent of women with PTSD also have postpartum depression, and 22% of women with postpartum depression also have PTSD (Grisbrook & Letourneau, 2021). Studies from other countries have also found PTSD to be highly comorbid with postpartum depression.

A longitudinal study of 206 Latinas in the US found that depressive symptoms predicted PTSD symptoms during pregnancy and at 7 and 13 months postpartum (Sumner et al., 2012). They were mostly low-income women from Mexico with low levels of acculturation. Risk factors for PTSD symptoms were low income, partner violence, childhood trauma, and low support at 7 months. Recent trauma, with co-occurring depression, was the best predictor of postpartum PTSD symptoms.

PTSD was highly comorbid with depression (73%), anxiety (64%), and moderate to high life stress (73%) in a study of 54 Caucasian, Asian, and Pacific Islander women with PTSD (Onoye et al., 2009). Although there were no significant differences in rates of PTSD based on ethnicity (possibly due to the small sample), Pacific Islanders had the highest rates of behavioral health problems.

A longitudinal study of 119 women in Hawai'i examined the change in symptoms of PTSD, depression, anxiety, and maternal stress during pregnancy and postpartum (Onoye et al., 2013). PTSD symptoms declined over the course of the pregnancy, with a spike in symptoms in the last weeks. Anxiety did not change for many over time; however, there was wide variability. These findings were consistent with previous studies showing more symptoms during pregnancy than postpartum.

In Shanghai, China, 24% of mothers were depressed and 6% had PTSD in a sample of 1,136 (Lui et al., 2021). PTSD was the strongest predictor for depression, and depression was the strongest predictor for PTSD. Low support, poor sleep quality, and non-Han ethnicity increased the risk of both. (Han was the dominant ethnicity.)

Eating Disorders

Eating disorders can also co-occur with depression during pregnancy and postpartum. In one study, active bulimia nervosa also increased the risk of postpartum depression, miscarriage, and preterm birth by 2 to 3 times (Morgan et al., 2006). In this study, a cohort of 122 pregnant women with active bulimia were compared with 82 pregnant women with quiescent bulimia. A population study of 1,119 women had a similar finding. Women with eating disorders had three times the risk for postpartum depression compared with women without eating disorders (Mazzeo et al., 2006). Concern over mistakes, a subtype of perfectionism, was related to more severe depression.

Substance Use

In a review of 17 studies, Ross and Dennis (2009) found that women who were actively using alcohol, cocaine, or other illegal drugs were at increased risk for postpartum depression. Substance use is obviously serious for both mothers and babies. If women use substances during pregnancy, the state may remove the baby from the mother's care after delivery. For substance-using mothers, intervention for depression alone would be incomplete. Mothers who use substances also need referrals to programs that can directly address their substance use.

Postpartum Psychosis

Postpartum psychosis is a rare form of postpartum mental illness that carries a high risk of both infanticide and suicide. It occurs in 0.1% to 0.2% of all new mothers, and most episodes begin abruptly within 10 to 14 days postpartum (Osborne, 2018). Early warning signs include insomnia, anxiety, irritability, and mood fluctuations.

Bipolar Disorder

Women's history of bipolar disorder is the single greatest risk factor for postpartum psychosis, and women with postpartum psychosis often develop bipolar disorder (Osborne, 2018), but psychosis can also occur in women with no prior history of mental health disorders. Postpartum bipolar disorder is often misdiagnosed because it first manifests as major depression. Mothers are then prescribed antidepressants, which can trigger manic episodes in those with underlying bipolar disorder. Symptoms of bipolar disorder include inflated self-esteem, increased talkativeness, decreased sleep, racing thoughts, and increased goal orientation. Mothers with bipolar disorder are 7 to 23 times more likely than mothers without bipolar disorder to be hospitalized (Clark & Wisner, 2018; Sharma et al., 2017).

The symptoms mothers experience can also vary depending on whether they have bipolar 1 or 2; the severity of the manic episodes differs by type. Bipolar 1 is more severe and causes full manic episodes, whereas bipolar 2 leads to less-severe hypomanic episodes. Differentiating major depression from bipolar disorder, particularly bipolar disorder 2, can be challenging. Hypomania is common during the postpartum period and is particularly common in women diagnosed with postpartum depression (Beck, 2006; Sharma et al., 2017; Yatham et al., 2009).

In a study of 30 women with bipolar disorders who had children, 66% were also depressed (Freeman et al., 2002). Most of these episodes were exclusively depressive. Of the women who became depressed after their first child, all were depressed after subsequent births. Depression during pregnancy also increased the risk of postpartum depression.

A study of 276 Italian women with bipolar disorder tracked their progress through the postpartum period (Maina et al., 2014). All had been medication-free throughout their pregnancies. Seventy-five percent had a history of postpartum mood disorders. Depression was the most common (80%), but 14% had had manic episodes, and 4% had mixed episodes. Thirteen patients had psychosis. Women with bipolar disorder that was unmedicated during pregnancy were at high risk for mood disorders and psychosis postpartum.

Birth can also trigger psychosis in bipolar women with a family history of postpartum psychosis (Jones & Craddock, 2001). These researchers examined 313 deliveries of 152 women with bipolar disorder. Twenty-six percent of the deliveries were followed by postpartum psychosis, and 38% of the women had at least one postpartum psychotic episode. In the 27 women with bipolar disorder who had a family history of postpartum psychosis, 74% developed postpartum psychosis. In contrast, only 30% of the women with bipolar disorder without a family history had postpartum psychosis.

Although bipolar has a strong genetic component, a review found that childhood trauma can also increase risk, noting that people with bipolar disorder have often experienced severe and frequent childhood trauma (Etain et al., 2008). Childhood trauma was associated with more severe symptoms and may affect the age of onset and suicidal behavior and comorbid depression, panic disorder, and substance use. It can also affect patients between episodes.

Antidepressants should be used cautiously due to the possible risk of inducing postpartum psychosis, mania, and rapid cycling (Freeman et al., 2002; Moses-Kolko & Roth, 2004). In published case reports, mania happened to those with a family history of bipolar disorder (Yatham et al., 2009). For these women, the anticonvulsant medications may be more appropriate in that they have both mood-stabilizing and antidepressant effects.

Sleep Deprivation and Psychosis

Severe sleep deprivation can cause psychotic symptoms in men and non-postpartum women. Severe sleeplessness can also proceed to psychosis in postpartum women. Women with psychosis who were interviewed for this book all indicated that they had been unable to sleep for two to three days before their psychotic break. **Inability to sleep not related to baby care is a red flag that requires immediate medical attention.** Charlotte describes her experience.

> My second postpartum experience was a nightmare. I was exhausted. . . . I decided to wean my baby at 2 months because I was so exhausted and depressed. . . . I thought about suicide, institutionalization, and separation from my family constantly. . . . That postpartum psychosis exists was such a revelation to me because in April I had experienced a week of near-total insomnia. During these truly sleepless nights, I had no control over my thoughts, as if my brain had been put in a food processor. The first half of a thought would be rational, and the second half would be totally unrelated, nonsensical.

The exact mechanism for the sleep-deprivation/psychosis link is unclear currently.

Clinical Takeaways

- Mothers who are depressed during pregnancy or postpartum have a high likelihood of having comorbid conditions.
- When clinicians only screen for depression, they will miss comorbid conditions, limiting the effectiveness of their treatment.
- Of the comorbid conditions, anxiety and PTSD are most common. But others may be present.
- A mother who has not slept in 2 or 3 days needs immediate medical attention. This is often a prodrome to postpartum psychosis.

Note

1 Pregnancy Risk Assessment Monitoring. A system used by the US Centers for Disease Control and Prevention.

2   Incidence of Depression in New Mothers and Fathers

The incidence of postpartum depression varies and depends on the study sample and how the authors have defined *depression*. I have estimated that the typical range is 12% to 25%, with rates in some high-risk groups being 50% or higher. A recent systematic review of 291 studies from 56 countries found a similar range (Hahn-Holbrook et al., 2018). This review included data from 296,284 women and found that the global pooled prevalence was 18% but ranged across studies from 3% to 28%. If the study used the Edinburgh Postnatal Depression Scale (EPDS) with a cutoff of 10 or higher, which also includes mild depression, prevalence was 21%. Using a more stringent cutoff of 13 or more that only includes more severe depression, the prevalence was 17%. Countries differed significantly based on income inequality, infant and maternal mortality, and if women with children worked 40 or more hours a week. These factors explained 73% of the variance. This chapter summarizes studies from around the world.

KEY FINDINGS

- International prevalence of postpartum depression is 21% if measures also included mild depression, and 17% if only severe depression was included.
- Recent studies reveal that racial/ethnic minority American women have higher rates of depression than their White counterparts, ranging from 15% to 30%
- Depression rates are also high at 4 to 5 years postpartum.
- Babies are protected from the effects of even war trauma if their mothers have good mental health.
- New fathers can also be depressed. Current studies indicate that their prevalence of depression is usually lower than that of mothers and often occurs for different reasons. One review estimated that prenatal depression affects 14 million fathers worldwide, and postpartum depression affects 12 million.
- When one partner is depressed, it increases risk for the other one.

United States

A recent study from the US Pregnancy Risk Assessment Monitoring System (PRAMS) included mothers from 31 sites. They found that 13.2% were depressed, but the rate varied by state, ranging from 10% in Illinois to 24% in Mississippi (Bauman et al., 2020). The Childbirth Connections' Listening to Mothers' II Survey found that depressive symptoms were common in a sample of 1,573 American mothers (Declercq et al., 2008). One

DOI: 10.4324/9781003411246-3

in three mothers reported depressive symptoms in the past two weeks: 34% reported feeling down, depressed, or hopeless, and 36% reported anhedonia (little interest or pleasure in doing things).

A longitudinal study from Baltimore found rates of depression increased from the first (12%) and second (14%) trimester to be highest in the last trimester (30%) (Setse et al., 2009). Nine percent were depressed postpartum. Depression was assessed using the Center for Epidemiologic Studies—Depression.

US Racial/Ethnic Minorities

In 2015, the US Centers for Disease Control and Prevention stated that younger women, African Americans, Hispanics, other non-White women were least likely to be diagnosed with and treated for depression (Centers for Disease Control and Prevention, 2015). There was a large gap in the literature regarding ethnic minority populations in Western countries. Fortunately, this is beginning to change, and there are new studies that are addressing the knowledge gap. Recent PRAMS data found that 11% of White women were depressed compared to 18% of Black women, 22% of American Indians or Alaska Natives, and 19% of Asian or Pacific Islanders (non-Hispanic) (Bauman et al., 2020).

In a prospective of 1,735 women, Mora and colleagues (2009) described the trajectories of depressive symptoms over 2 years in a sample of low-income, multiethnic, inner-city women. Seventy percent of the women were African American, 17% were Latina, and the remaining 13% were White, Asian, or other ethnicities. Twenty-nine percent were depressed either during pregnancy or postpartum, and a further 15% had transient symptoms. Based on their analyses, women fell into five distinct groups: chronically depressed (7%); prenatal depression only (6%); postpartum only—resolves in the first year postpartum (9%); late-presenting depression at 25 months (7%); and never having depression (71%).

A recent scoping review of 9 articles found that American Indian/Alaska Native (AI/AN) women were at increased risk for depression (Heck, 2021). Eleven percent of all women in the US have postpartum depression. In contrast, the prevalence for AI/AN women ranged from 14% to 30%, which was the highest. Cultural trauma was also cited as a factor. The author noted significant gaps in the literature and few studies on Alaska Native women. Further, many of the studies did not use a validated depression screening tool and assessed depression with a single yes/no question.

Focus groups of 133 Spanish-speaking Latina mothers described their experiences with postpartum depression; 28% of participants had given birth in the previous year (Sampson et al., 2021). The mothers described *familismo*, the cultural belief that encourages loyalty to family above all, which is generally a protective factor. Yet these mothers suggested that it can also increase their risk for depression. According to *familismo*, mothers are the "glue" of their families. They are expected to sacrifice and suffer for their children. In this sample, 23% to 51% of the mothers were depressed. Depression isolated them and made them feel useless to their families. Mothers wanted to lean on their families and community for help but felt that people were judging them, so they kept their feelings to themselves. In addition, Latina mothers who had recently immigrated were less likely to have the family and community support that they would have had in their home countries, which also increased their risk for depression.

A meta-analysis of 6 published studies examined postpartum depression in Indigenous mothers from Australia, Canada, New Zealand, and the US (Black et al., 2019).

Data were limited, but existing studies suggested a "greater burden of PPD affecting Indigenous women." They found that Indigenous women were 1.87 times more likely to be diagnosed with postpartum women than White women. Maori women from New Zealand were twice as likely to be depressed compared to White women, and American Indian women were 70% more likely to be depressed.

Europe

A Spanish study screened 1,453 mothers for psychiatric disorders. Eighteen percent had at least one, with mood disorders being the most common (Navarro et al., 2008). The combination of depression and anxiety was the most common, but eating disorders and depression were also common.

In Turkey, a study of 479 pregnant women found a similar rate: 18% in the first week postpartum and 14% at 6 weeks (Kirpinar et al., 2010). A second study from Turkey had similar results (Turkcapar et al., 2015), and 15% (*n* = 83) were depressed. Women who thought about suicide during pregnancy were seven times more likely to have postpartum depression.

Australia

A community-based online survey from Australia (*n* = 1,070) found that 13.4% of mothers had anxiety and depression (Ramakrishna et al., 2019). Women were more likely to have comorbid depression if they had financial problems, inadequate social support, and babies with difficult temperaments who also slept poorly. Mothers with depression and anxiety were 86% more likely to not be breastfeeding and were more likely to report their health as fair or poor, compared to mothers without anxiety and depression.

A 5-year longitudinal study of 343 women assessed depression, anxiety, and stress in 343 women who were experiencing adversity (Bryson et al., 2021). Mental health symptoms were highest during pregnancy and at 4 to 5 years postpartum. To be included in the study, mothers had to have experienced at least 2 adversities that included young pregnancy, not living with another adult, no support during pregnancy, poor health, long-term illness or disability, current smoking, stress, anxiety, difficulty coping, low education, no person in the household earning a living, and never having had a job before. The percentage of women experiencing high mental health problems was 20% to 30% over the 5-year period. Women experiencing adversity had twice the rate of depression compared to the general population. The authors also noted that high rates of depression at 5 years are frequently ignored.

Another Australian study had similar findings: the highest rates of depression were at 4 years postpartum (Woolhouse et al., 2015). This study recruited 1,507 women during pregnancy from six Melbourne public hospitals. The mothers were assessed 5 times up to 4 years postpartum. The study revealed that 31% of women had depressive symptoms at some time in the first 4 years postpartum. Women with one child at 4 years postpartum had significantly higher rates of depression (23%) than women with more than one child (11%). In the first 12 months, the strongest predictors were young maternal age, stressful life events, social adversity, intimate partner violence, and low income.

Asia

A review of 64 studies from 17 countries in Asia found that postpartum depression varied widely, ranging from 3.5% in Malaysia to 63% in Pakistan (Klainin & Arthur, 2009). In Asian cultures, depression is often manifested as somatic symptoms. This review included Russia, Turkey, and the Middle East as part of Asia so is broader than most reviews. Risk factors were similar to those in Western cultures: lack of support, low income, violence, and breastfeeding difficulties.

A study of 153 women from Korea found that the prevalence of depression ranged from 41% to 61% (Park et al., 2015). They evaluated women during pregnancy and at 4 weeks postpartum. Murray and colleagues (Murray et al., 2015) compared urban (n = 216) and rural (n = 215) samples from Central Vietnam. They examined the impact of son preference, traditional confinement practices, poverty, parity, infant health, partner violence, and infant health on postpartum depression. Twenty percent of the urban women and 16% of the rural women had depressive symptoms. Infant sex was not related to depression, but poverty, food insecurity, breastfeeding difficulties, being frightened of family members, mother-in-law reacting negatively to the baby, and recent partner violence were. Regarding traditional confinement practices, mothers had less depression if they were *not* practiced. Mothers were less depressed if they were able to watch TV, could bathe, wash their hair, read, and if they avoided eating special foods. Only using traditional medicine resulted in lower depression scores.

A longitudinal study of 160 Chinese women found that depression ranged from 26% to 35% (from pregnancy to postpartum), and anxiety ranged from 53% to 64% (Cheng et al., 2021). Depression, anxiety, and stress were strongly correlated. Depression and anxiety rose during pregnancy and were highest postpartum. In contrast, stress followed a different pattern: it dropped during pregnancy but rose again postpartum.

South America

Twenty-nine percent of 227 women from Brazil were depressed postpartum, and depression and anxiety were positively correlated (Silva et al., 2021). Women with moderate anxiety were 17 times more likely to develop depression. Eighteen percent had suicidal ideations.

Middle East

In a prospective study of 137 women from the United Arab Emirates, 17% had depressive symptoms and 10% were formally diagnosed with depression at 2 months postpartum (Hamdan & Tamim, 2011). Non-Arabic women were excluded from the sample. The factors that predicted postpartum depression were depression in pregnancy, number of children, non-Muslim religion, and formula feeding. (Non-Muslims were religious minorities in the UAE.)

A study of 511 pregnant women from the Gaza strip assessed them during pregnancy and at 4 and 12 months postpartum. The mothers reported PTSD, depressive, anxiety, and dissociative symptoms (Punamaki et al., 2018). War trauma did not directly affect infant outcomes. However, there was an indirect effect of war trauma via mothers' mental health during pregnancy and postpartum. Mothers' depression, anxiety, or

PTSD predicted poor outcomes for infants' sensorimotor and language development at 12 months. War trauma also increased the risk of pregnancy complications. These findings suggest that interventions targeting maternal mental health will improve infant outcomes. The authors recommended strengthening mothers' sense of security, their interactions with their babies, and their access to psychosocial support. They noted that "horrors of war do not impact children's well-being and development if mothers are able to maintain their good mental health" (p. 151).

Another study compared women in two rural communities in Pakistan (*n* = 1,727) and Malawi (*n* = 1,732) and found marked differences in "postpartum psychological morbidity": 27% in Pakistan and 3% in Malawi (Zafar et al., 2015). The rates of depression could differ based on where the data were collected (in home setting in Pakistan vs busy clinic in Malawi). In addition, women in Malawi were more involved in agricultural or other work and not confined to home. In Malawi (and other African cultures), admitting to anxiety or worry may be associated with "wishing it upon yourself," so disclosure rates are likely to be lower. Finally, mothers in Malawi may experience more support that prevents depression and anxiety from occurring.

Africa

In the Sudan, a sample of 300 pregnant women were enrolled in a study, and 238 participated at 3 months postpartum (Khalifa et al., 2015). Nine percent had postpartum depression. The percentage of depressed women is surprisingly low, given the ongoing civil war and major social disruptions. The authors recommended assessing depression after 6 weeks postpartum because mothers in the first 6 weeks receive intense social support. Could this intense support prevent depression even in severe circumstances?

More recent African studies found higher rates. In Nigeria, a study of 250 new mothers found that 37% were depressed (Adeyemo et al., 2020). Multiparity, cesarean delivery, being unwell after birth, and not exclusively breastfeeding were related to depression. Postpartum blues increased risk by 32 times; no help with the baby and an unsupportive partner by 2.6 times. Regarding breastfeeding, 77% of formula-feeding mothers were depressed, compared to 40% of mixed-feeding mothers, and 31% of those who were exclusively breastfeeding.

A study of 200 mothers from Nairobi, Kenya, found that 13% were depressed (Madeghe et al., 2016). The authors were particularly interested in the link between depression and child malnutrition and stunted growth, and they specifically targeted Nairobi because the child malnutrition rate is high. Non-depressed mothers were 6.14 times more likely to exclusively breastfeed. Babies of depressed mothers were 4.4 times more likely to be underweight. Of the 27% of women who supplemented, only 8% used formula. The most common supplements were water and soft porridge. Some mothers had a low milk supply because they did not have enough to eat.

A study from Northern Ethiopia of 596 postpartum mothers found that 24% were depressed (Shitu et al., 2019). Most of the women in this sample were farmers, and two-thirds had no formal education. There was no relationship between substance use and depression. In contrast, a study of 456 postpartum women (up to 12 months) from Southwest Ethiopia found that substance use increased the risk of depression by more than 5 times (Toru et al., 2018). The prevalence of postpartum depression was 22%. Previous depression was the strongest risk factor, increasing risk by 7.38 times. Regarding demographics, 35% of husbands had a diploma, and 52% were merchants.

Depression in New Fathers

An increasing number of researchers are finding depression in new fathers. These findings may also be relevant to same-sex partners, but studies specific to them are lacking so far. A recent review notes the paucity of this research (Darwin et al., 2021). If mothers are depressed, fathers are also likely to be depressed. Women are at higher risk for depression early in the postpartum period. In contrast, men's depression begins later and increases more gradually. Men are also less likely to seek help (Letourneau et al., 2012). Men and women who are depressed can have similar symptoms, but men's symptoms are more likely to be anxiety or anger rather than sadness. Men may also be indecisive, cynical, or irritable (Melrose, 2010). In addition, the external stressors leading to depression often differ. Relationship difficulties can be both a cause and a consequence of depression, particularly when both partners are affected.

A study from Canada compared fathers with and without depression (de Montigny et al., 2013). The infants in the study were exclusively breastfeeding. Risk factors for fathers' depression included previous perinatal loss, child with a difficult temperament, and perceived low parental efficacy.

A longitudinal study of 200 couples from Hong Kong showed that high levels of depressive symptoms during pregnancy, and partner's depressive symptoms, significantly increased fathers' depressive symptoms at 6 months postpartum (Ngai & Ngu, 2015). The prevalence rate for fathers was 7% during pregnancy, and 11% at 6 months postpartum. The prevalence rate for mothers was 16% during pregnancy, and 13% at 6 months postpartum. Lack of social support was a depression risk factor for mothers, but not for fathers. A survey from Japan of 837 new parents found that 14% of fathers and 10% of mothers were depressed (Nishimura et al., 2015). For fathers, the risk factors included a history of infertility treatment, going to a medical facility for treatment of a mental disorder, and economic anxiety.

A screening study from Sweden found that 8% of fathers had postpartum depression, and 89% were willing to accept treatment (Asper et al., 2018). Similarly, a meta-analysis of 74 studies with 41,480 participants found that 8.4% of fathers across studies had paternal depression (Cameron et al., 2016). However, the authors noted "significant heterogeneity" among the reported prevalence rates. These rates were influenced by study year and location, measure used, and maternal depression. Factors not associated with fathers' depression were age, education, parity, history of depression, or timing of the assessment. They found that North America had the highest rates of depressed fathers, almost 13%, while Europe and Australia had the lowest rates. Most of the North American studies were from the US. The authors speculated that this might be due to lack of paid leave in the US. Fathers were at highest risk for depression at 3 to 6 months postpartum.

A longitudinal study of 126 Italian fathers analyzed trajectories of depression from pregnancy to 1 year postpartum (Molgora et al., 2017). The researchers identified three patterns of depression over time in these fathers: low symptoms (resilient: 52%); moderate, stable depressive symptoms (distress: 37%); and high depressive symptoms (emergent depression: 11%). These findings indicate that 48% of fathers in this study had moderate to severe depressive symptoms.

A meta-analysis of 47 studies (*n* = 20,728) of prenatal depression in fathers worldwide found a prevalence of 10% (Rao et al., 2020). It ranged from 14% in the first trimester, 11% in the second, and 10% in the third trimester. Nine percent were depressed over the first year. Their results suggested that 14 million fathers worldwide were depressed prenatally, and 12 million had postpartum depression.

Anxiety also appears to be more common in men during the perinatal period than at other times. A meta-analysis of 23 studies (*n* = 40,124) found that 11% had prenatal and postpartum anxiety, but there was significant heterogeneity between the samples (Leiferman et al., 2021).

Causes of Fathers' Depression

A prospective study from Northern Iran examined mothers' and fathers' prenatal and postpartum depression (Barooj-Kiakalaee et al., 2022). Mothers' depression directly and indirectly affected fathers' depression. In Japan, a sample of fathers at 1 month (*n* = 1,023) and 6 months (*n* = 1,330) found that 11% to 12% of fathers were depressed (Nishigori et al., 2020). At one month, risk factors included history of mental disorders, distress during pregnancy, and infant illness that required treatment. At 6 months, risk factors included distress during pregnancy, unemployment, and maternal postpartum depression.

A qualitative study from Sweden explored possible reasons for fathers to be depressed (Johansson et al., 2020). Fifteen mothers and fathers participated in the study. Mothers and fathers felt inadequate, but the source of their inadequacy differed: internal requirements for mothers (responsibilities of caring for their families) vs external requirements for fathers (demanding work schedule, childcare restrictions, the economy). Traumatic childbirth affected both, as did spouse relationship problems. Childhood adversity or previous trauma increased the risk of depression for mothers, but not fathers.

Another qualitative study of 8 fathers found that fatherhood was an overwhelming experience (Pedersen et al., 2021). They felt inadequate and powerless related to their expected role as fathers to be, which made them angry and frustrated. A meta-analysis of 47 studies on fathers also identified challenges of caring for a newborn, including sleepless nights and feeding difficulties, mothers' mental health, and increased expenses and the economic burden of caring for an infant (Rao et al., 2020).

Quality of their sleep was another important risk factor for fathers and was assessed for 2 weeks in a study of 54 fathers at 6 months postpartum (Kalogerpoulos et al., 2021). Sleep diary variables, such as total sleep time and number of nighttime awakenings, were not related to depression. Similarly, objective sleep measures were not related to depression. However, if fathers reported that their sleep quality was poor, they were more likely to be depressed.

A meta-analysis of 17 cross-sectional studies indicated that fathers' unemployment, history of mothers' mental illness, first pregnancy, and poor marital relationship were related to postpartum depression in fathers (Wang et al., 2021). If fathers had a history of mental illness, it increased their risk by 3.48 times. Unemployment increased risk by 2.59 times, and financial strain by 2.07 times. Surprisingly, mothers' postpartum depression only slightly increased risk. Nine of the studies found that infant characteristics and preference for a male infant were the factors most strongly related to depression.

Clinical Takeaways

- Postpartum depression affects mothers and fathers from a broad range of backgrounds, ethnicities, and nationalities.

- Rates are higher in countries with higher infant or maternal mortality, war, or significant poverty.
- Racial/ethnic mothers in the US may be particularly at risk.
- Fathers are also at risk for depression and anxiety. Some studies found that mothers' mental health was a risk factor for fathers' depression, but not all studies found this. Other risk factors were sleep problems and issues related to them being the family provider.

3 Depression's Negative Impact on Mothers

Depression and other mental health disorders can harm those who experience it. A review of 24 studies found that mental health disorders doubled the risk of premature mortality worldwide and shortened life by a median of 10 years (Walker et al., 2015). Eight million deaths per year can be attributed to mental health disorders. Depression increases the risk of coronary heart disease, myocardial infarction, chronic pain syndromes, premature aging, impaired wound healing, and even Alzheimer's disease (Kiecolt-Glaser et al., 2005). Postpartum depression is also harmful. This chapter summarizes general health effects of depression and two particularly salient potential harms: suicidal ideations and suicide. Ongoing postpartum depression has the same detrimental physical effect as depression in the general population.

KEY FINDINGS

- Approximately 15% of new mothers think about suicide.
- Suicide is relatively rare, but one study found that 49% of mothers seeking treatment for postpartum mental illness had attempted it.

Health and Well-Being

According to the US Centers for Disease Control and Prevention, depression affects women's lives in many ways, including their family relationships, their ability to function at home or at work, and their future risk of chronic disease, including diabetes and heart disease (Centers for Disease Control and Prevention, 2015). A review of 61 studies focused specifically on the consequences of postpartum depression and found that it negatively affected physical health and quality of life (Slomian et al., 2019). Depressed women are less likely to use contraception, or to use less-effective forms, and are more likely to smoke, have high BMIs, and use emergency medical services. They are also more likely to binge-drink or drink heavily. Unfortunately, 66% of women who were depressed during pregnancy were not diagnosed (Centers for Disease Control and Prevention, 2015).

Inflammation is behind many physical illnesses, including heart disease and diabetes (see Chapter 5). Not surprisingly, because inflammation is already high in people with these conditions, they are at higher risk for depression (de Jonge et al., 2006; Preston, 2022). For example, an epidemiological study (n = 18,109) found that women with gestational diabetes mellitus (GDM) had significantly higher risk for postpartum depression and anxiety (Walmer et al., 2015). Hispanic women with gestational diabetes were at highest risk, followed by White, Asian, and Black women. Black women with gestational

DOI: 10.4324/9781003411246-4

diabetes had higher rates of depression compared to Black women who did not have it. Higher income lessened this effect. Thirty-four percent of women with gestational diabetes had depressive symptoms at 6 weeks postpartum in a sample of 71 women (Nicklas et al., 2013). Cesarean delivery and higher weight gain during pregnancy increased the risk of depression.

Suicidal Ideations

Sometimes, while depressed, women think about hurting or killing themselves. The exact percentage is not known since women are unlikely to disclose this information. But studies suggest that thoughts of suicide are more common than we have previously believed.

Self-Harm and Suicidal Ideations

A longitudinal study of 1,507 women from pregnancy to 4 years postpartum found that 4% to 5% thought about harming themselves at each time point, but these ideations were most common in the first 12 months (Giallo et al., 2018). Fifteen percent thought about harming themselves but were not thinking about dying. Thoughts of self-harm increased if mothers were depressed during pregnancy and early postpartum, were unemployed while pregnant, lacked social support the first year, and had experienced childhood physical abuse.

A study of 147 Canadian postpartum women found that 17% reported thoughts of self-harm, and 6% reported suicidal ideation in the first year (Pope et al., 2013). The sample included women with major depression and bipolar disorder II. Women who were more depressed were more likely to think about suicide. Women with hypomanic symptoms were at highest risk.

An Italian study measured suicidality during pregnancy and at 12 months postpartum in a sample of 1,066 women (Mauri et al., 2012). "Suicidality" was defined as "thoughts of death or self-harm and suicide attempts." Five hundred women completed the assessment at 12 months. For the whole sample, the point prevalence for suicidality ranged from 7% to 12% during pregnancy, and 4% to 12% postpartum. For depressed women, the suicidality rate ranged from 26% to 34% during pregnancy, and 18% to 31% postpartum. Four mothers I've interviewed indicated that they too had suicidal ideations.

- I'm still dealing with sexual abuse [her own history]. I hadn't dealt with it before the birth. I told my husband for the first time in the hospital. I was hysterical. . . I was afraid of being alone, so my husband stayed the night. If I could've opened the window, I would have jumped out.
- I had breastfeeding problems. He was colicky. I was afraid I wouldn't be able to comfort him. I didn't have thoughts of hurting him, but I thought of suicide. That's how depressed I was.
- The severe depression would come on and go away. One time I was sorting through all our medicines, sorting the ones that were very lethal into a pile. The severe episodes only lasted about 1/2 a minute, but the moderate depression stayed. I couldn't be left alone.
- My husband and sister thought they would take care of me. I started having visions of my own funeral. I was having all kinds of scary thoughts. At that point, they decided I needed to go into the hospital. . . The week after my daughter's birthday, I was

acutely suicidal. I packed some clothes and my pills. I was going to go to New York City, rent a hotel room, and kill myself. My husband said I was rambling and saying, "Please take care of her." As I was getting on the train, my husband was at the train station because they found my car.

A study from Bangladesh (n = 361) found that 33% were depressed (Gausia et al., 2009). The strongest risk factors for depression were being beaten by their husbands before or during their pregnancies, no support from their husbands or mothers-in-law, and preferring a male child. If they were depressed while pregnant, 14% thought of self-harm. The mothers often felt that they had no way out of their current situation. Twenty percent could not read and had never been to school, and another 25% had only been to school for 1 to 5 years. Most were not employed, and they could not return to their families because of the shame that it would bring upon them.

Some mothers have both suicidal thoughts and thoughts of infant harm. Valerie first developed thoughts about the baby being hurt, then her hurting the baby. She also thought about ending her own life. She had a family history of severe depression and a personal history of miscarriage and infertility. Her symptoms were severe enough for her to talk to her midwife.

My husband and I tried for 4 years to get pregnant. During that time, we had two miscarriages: one at 6 weeks and one at 10 weeks. When we finally did get pregnant, I stifled my excitement till about the third trimester because I was sure something was going to happen, and my son was going to die.

I hadn't even had a problem with depression myself, so I was not prepared for it when it hit me after the baby was born. I didn't think it would happen to me because I wanted to have a baby so badly. About a week after my son was born, I started having horrible images pop into my head of me hurting my son. They started out as images of accidents happening: me dropping him accidentally on the pavement. But by the time he was a month and a half old, they turned into images of me doing things on purpose to him, like walking into the corner of the wall and hitting his head on the corner until he was unconscious. I specifically remember one night, in particular, I had nursed my son to sleep, and then laid him on my chest and rocked him. I was in a little nook area right next to my kitchen, and I went from enjoying my baby to suddenly having the urge to grab a knife and put it through my baby's back and into my heart. It took everything I had in me to stop myself from doing it. Once I was able to dismiss the desire to end both of our precious lives, I got up away from the knives and found my husband. I didn't have the courage to tell him why, but I told him I was going to talk to the midwife about postpartum depression at my 6-week appointment that week.

My wonderful midwife talked to me about my depression. She didn't ask for specifics, bless her soul, because I wasn't ready to talk about them just yet. I felt so guilty for the thoughts I had that I thought it would be better for the baby if I just left him and his dad. I didn't know what I would do once I left, but I didn't think I should have the privilege of being in my baby's life.

My midwife put me on Prozac and sent me to a psychiatrist (who was amazing). She helped me realize that all these thoughts of harming myself and my baby were the depression talking, and that it wasn't my fault. It just happens to some women.

I had, and still have, lots of people rooting for me, and I am very grateful for all their support and love.

Suicidality can also affect mothers' interactions with their babies. A study of 32 mothers found that suicidality causes cognitive distortions where mothers believe that they are the "worst mothers in the world," and that their babies would be better off without them (Anda et al., 2009). Suicidality made these mothers less sensitive to their infants' cues and social signals and limited their ability to respond consistently. The infants responded with less positive affect and were less engaged in the interactions. The authors speculated that these mothers might believe that they were "toxic" for their babies and distanced themselves from their babies to protect them.

Suicide

Suicide is the leading cause of death in postpartum women (Aronsson et al., 2015). It is, fortunately, relatively rare, but suicide attempts are more common. In a sample from Liverpool, UK, of 73 mothers referred to a perinatal mental health clinic, 49% had made a probable suicide attempt (Healey et al., 2013).

Suicide leaves behind a heartbroken family. Depression activist Joan Mudd writes, "In 2001 my dear daughter, Jennifer Mudd Houghtaling, lost her battle with postpartum depression." A tribute to Jennifer described her as follows.

No one would be more stunned by the turn of events that created the Jennifer Mudd Houghtaling Postpartum Depression Foundation than Jennifer. Her ebullient joy, and laser beam of personal interest and insight, were her gifts to everyone she knew and loved. Carefree, energetic, devoted, and nonjudgmental, Jennifer would want to know what she could do to help this cause, how does this terrible disease occur, and most of all, what needs to be done to solve it.

It was her generosity of spirit that was so special. . . Jennifer made all those around her feel like they mattered.

That light should have shone brightly on her much desired and cherished baby boy, Brandon. More than anything, Jennifer wanted Brandon. When she found out that she was carrying a baby boy, she named him immediately, and changed the password on her computer to Brandon so she could see his name and say it every day.

In 2004, Joan and her husband founded the Jennifer Mudd Houghtaling Foundation to increase awareness of postpartum depression among healthcare providers, increase screening for new mothers, and save other women from what happened to Jennifer.

Clinical Takeaways

- Depressed new mothers think about harming or killing themselves more often than we have previously believed.
- All mothers and fathers with postpartum mental illness should be screened for suicide risk.

4 Maternal Depression Negatively Affects Babies and Children

Mothers' depression harms them and can potentially harm their children. Fortunately, many things modify this potential harm, but it is there. I write this chapter not to heap more guilt on mothers; rather, my goal is underscore depression's seriousness, hoping that it will be identified and treated quickly. While most of this research has focused on mothers' depression, fathers' depression can also affect their children. To date, we have no studies on same-sex partners, but I believe that future studies will find a similar effect. Without intervention, postpartum depression has serious, long-lasting negative consequences for infants. Hoping that it will get better on its own is magical thinking and is never a viable option.

KEY FINDINGS

- Depression, anxiety, and PTSD increase the risk for preterm birth, the second leading cause of infant mortality worldwide.
- Long-chain omega-3 fatty acids (EPA and DHA) and social support decrease the risk of preterm birth because they lower inflammation.
- Mothers' prenatal or postpartum depression sensitizes infants' stress responses to stressful or novel situations. Breastfeeding appears to mediate this effect.
- Maternal depression, anxiety, or PTSD are related to poorer developmental outcomes than in infants of mothers without mental illness.
- Untreated mental illness likely harms babies because it affects the way that parents interact with them. Babies of depressed parents are less likely to form a secure attachment, which affects many aspects of development.
- Prenatal and postpartum depression increase the risk of obesity in preschoolers and school-aged children.
- Mothers' prenatal and postpartum depression increase amygdala volume of their school-aged children. Higher volume indicates distress.
- Maternal and paternal depression predicts higher rates of smoking, substance use, major depression, and anxiety in young adult offspring.
- Depression influences mothers' interaction style with their infants. They are more likely to disengage and have flat affect, which raises babies' cortisol.
- Several studies have found increased cortisol reactivity in offspring of depressed mothers, which has potentially serious implications for the offspring's physical and mental health.
- Depressed breastfeeding mothers cannot fully disengage from their infants. This was enough to protect infants from the effects of their mothers' depression.

DOI: 10.4324/9781003411246-5

The Impact of Untreated Prenatal Depression on Preterm Birth and Infant Mortality

Depression, anxiety, and PTSD during pregnancy are potentially lethal for babies because they increase the risk for preterm birth, the second leading cause of infant mortality worldwide (Centers for Disease Control, 2019). That alone should urge people to screen pregnant women, but practitioners are often lax because they do not understand the serious consequences. I hope to demonstrate in this section why screening for and addressing these conditions are critical. Anecdotally, I learned that the rate of preterm birth was markedly increased during COVID-19. I suspect the rise is due to the same mechanism which I describe in Chapter 5. Fortunately, there are some simple preventative things mothers can do to lower their risk.

Depression and Preterm Birth

A study of 261 African American women found that depression increased the risk for preterm birth, low birthweight, and preeclampsia (Kim et al., 2013). Thirty-five percent were depressed. Another study of African American pregnant women (*n* = 1,270) found that 20% were depressed and that depression increased the risk for preterm birth by 70% (Nutor et al., 2018). A systematic review of 39 articles concluded that there was "strong evidence" that depression, anxiety, and stress during pregnancy increase the risk of preterm birth (Staneva et al., 2015).

The link between depression, pregnancy and preterm birth is true worldwide. A review of 29 studies found that prenatal depression increased risk of preterm birth and low birthweight (Grote et al., 2010). The risk was greater for women in developing countries than in North America or Europe. Their calculations revealed that prenatal depression was comparable to smoking 10 or more cigarettes a day. However, antenatal depression had less risk than Black race and using substances. The combined risk of Black race and antenatal depression would be higher still. Further, there was a cumulative effect of adversities, such as depression, living in poverty, facing discrimination, and experiencing food insecurity.

Anxiety Disorders and Preterm Birth

Anxiety can also increase the risk of preterm birth. A study of 1,820 women from Baltimore found that women who were anxious about their pregnancies had significantly more preterm babies (Orr, 2007). These findings were true even after controlling for other risk factors, including race/ethnicity, first- or second-trimester bleeding, drug use, unemployment, previous preterm birth or stillbirth, smoking, and low BMI, maternal education, and age.

Another study of 415 pregnant women from LA had similar results (Glynn et al., 2008). The sample was 23% Hispanic, 48% White, 14% African American, and 15% of women from other ethnic groups. Higher stress and anxiety increased the risk of preterm birth. These findings persisted even after controlling for obstetric risk, pregnancy-related anxiety, race/ethnicity, parity, and prenatal life events. More recently, a review and meta-analysis of 29 studies found that anxiety during pregnancy increased risk for preterm birth, low birthweight, earlier gestational age, small for gestational age, and smaller head circumference (Grigoriadis et al., 2018).

Posttraumatic Stress Disorder and Preterm Birth

A study of 2,654 pregnant women in Massachusetts and Connecticut examined the link between depression, PTSD, use of benzodiazepines and SSRIs, and preterm birth (Yonkers et al., 2014). PTSD was independently related to preterm birth. However, risk increased by 4 times if a mother had both PTSD and depression, independent of medication use. Prior child sexual abuse increased the risk, and one prior preterm birth quadrupled the risk. The researchers hypothesized that trauma increased levels of the stress hormone CRH, which serves as a "placental clock." Too much CRH tells the body it's time to have the baby. Inflammation is another possible mechanism. Two proinflammatory cytokines that are high in depression, anxiety, and PTSD, IL-6 and TNF-α, also ripen the cervix (Coussons-Read et al., 2005). (See Chapter 5.)

A study compared three groups of pregnant women: trauma-exposed, PTSD+ ($n = 255$); trauma-exposed, PTSD- ($n = 307$); and non-exposed ($n = 277$) (Seng et al., 2011). Twenty-two percent of the PTSD+ group had preterm babies, with 13% being low birthweight. Generally, researchers consider lower income and African American race to be the two strongest predictors of preterm birth. However, PTSD related to child sexual abuse was a stronger predictor of gestation length than income or African American race.

A study of 16,334 deliveries at Veterans Affairs hospitals from 2000 to 2012 found the rate of preterm birth varied based on PTSD status (Shaw et al., 2014). In this sample, 7.4% of women with no PTSD had preterm infants compared to 8% who had prior PTSD. For women with current PTSD, the rate was 9.2%.

Inflammation and Preterm Birth

Inflammation underlies depression, anxiety, chronic stress, and PTSD and is likely the physiological mechanism that increases the risk of preterm birth. I describe this in more detail in Chapter 5, but for now, I describe inflammation's role in preterm birth. As one recent review states, "human studies have implicated IL-1, TNF, and IL-6 as major players in PTB [preterm birth]" (Cappelletti et al., 2016). These are the specific molecules that are high in depression.

A recent study examined cortisol levels and pro- and anti-inflammatory cytokines during the 3rd trimester of pregnancy for 96 pregnant women. The study compared cortisol and cytokine levels for low-income minority women and affluent Caucasian women (Corwin et al., 2013). They found higher cortisol in lower-income and racial/ethnic-minority women. In addition, the normal mechanism that turns off the inflammation response was active in affluent White women but not there for lower-income or minority women. Chronic stress in the low-SES/minority women can cause cortisol resistance, which limited their bodies' ability to control inflammation. Elevated inflammation increased their risk of preterm birth.

Coussons-Read and colleagues' (2012) study of 173 women found that those who had preterm babies had more general and pregnancy-related stress and higher IL-6 and TNF-α compared with women who delivered at term. The sample was 66% Latina. The rate of preterm birth was 11%. The researchers noted that prenatal stress, as marked by the increase in proinflammatory cytokines, shortens gestation.

Anti-Inflammatory Methods That Decrease Risk of Preterm Birth

Fortunately, there are some simple techniques that can lower risk of preterm birth by lowering inflammation. I describe treatment in Volume 2, but there is some urgency to mention these options that, potentially, could save babies' lives.

Long-Chain Omega-3 Fatty Acids

Long-chain omega-3 fatty acids are the first method that lowers risk of preterm birth. Long-chain omega-3 fatty acids include eicosapentaenoic acid (EPA) and docosahexaenoic acid (DHA), which are usually given as fish oil supplements. These fatty acids are often low in people who do not eat a lot of fish, and they specifically lower inflammation. People with high EPA and DHA have low levels of IL-1α and IL-1β, IL-6, and TNF-α, the inflammatory molecules responsible for depression (Ferrucci et al., 2006). An ingenuous population study found that in countries where people eat a lot of fish, they are less likely to have postpartum depression (Hibbeln, 2002).

DHA also increases gestation length. In a randomized trial that included 291 low-income mothers from Kansas City, mothers were randomized to eat one egg a day for the last trimester of their pregnancies (Smuts, 2003). The eggs were either normal or contained 133 mg of DHA. This is not a large dose and is under the recommended minimum of DHA, which is 200 mg/day (Kendall-Tackett, 2010). Even with this low dose, this simple intervention increased gestation by an average of 6 days.

A study from Australia of 2,399 pregnant women randomized mothers to receive 800 mg of DHA or a placebo from 21 weeks' gestation to birth (Makrides et al., 2010). The authors hoped to find lower depression in the mothers and higher infant IQ at 18 months. They found neither. However, women supplemented with DHA were more likely to be induced or have cesareans because they were *post-dates*.

The most convincing evidence is from a Cochrane Review of 70 RCTs ($n = 19,927$) on omega-3 supplementation during pregnancy. The review concluded that "omega-3 supplementation during pregnancy is an effective strategy for reducing the incidence of preterm birth" (Middleton et al., 2018). They concluded that more studies are not needed at this stage.

Social Support

Social support is another anti-inflammatory method for reducing the risk of preterm birth. A meta-analysis of 41 studies ($n = 73,037$) found that social support and integration significantly lowered levels of inflammation (Uchino et al., 2018). With regards to preterm birth, a study from Los Angeles compared 1,027 preterm births to 1,282 full-term births in a retrospective case-control study (Ghosh et al., 2010). Sixty-five percent of the mothers were Hispanic. Thirty-seven percent of the women reported moderate stress, and 14% reported high chronic stress. Social support lowered the risk of preterm birth. Conversely, for mothers with moderate to high stress, low support doubled the risk. Women reporting low support and/or high chronic stress were more likely to be young, with low levels of education, Black or US-born Latina, single, and low income.

Effects of Maternal Depression on Infants

After babies are born, mothers' emotional state affects the way they interact with their infants, which can influence babies' growth and development. A recent review of 74 articles found that mothers' postpartum stress, depression, and anxiety negatively affected their infants' developmental outcomes (Oyentunji & Chandra, 2020). Mothers' mental illness was related to infants' stunted growth, poor language and cognitive development, poor gross and fine motor movement, and sleep problems. However, breastfeeding modified these negative effects, and breastfeeding mothers had lower risk of depression. Further, when mothers had high breastfeeding efficacy, their infants had better developmental outcomes. (See also Chapter 6.)

Similarly, a review of 67 studies found that mothers' depression increased the risk of significant health effects during infancy (Slomian et al., 2019). Maternal depression was related to lower infant weight gain with higher adiposity, shorter length, and more illness in infancy. Three out of 7 studies showed impaired motor development from ages 3 to 18 months.

Abnormal electroencephalogram (EEG) findings have been found in infants of depressed mothers at 3 to 6 months. Babies of depressed mothers had depressed affect and an EEG pattern that was similar to those of chronically depressed adults (right frontal EEG asymmetry) as early as 3 months (Field et al., 2006).

Emotional Regulation and Reactivity

Infants of depressed mothers are often more easily stressed. A study of 91 Portuguese women assessed them at 3 months before birth and 3 months after (Figueiredo & Costa, 2009). In the third trimester of pregnancy, 25% had anxiety or depression. At 3 months postpartum, 15% had anxiety and 27% were depressed. Mothers' depression predicted poorer prenatal attachment, but these mothers still had positive interactions with their infants. Conversely, mothers' anxiety did not affect prenatal attachment, but it did predict worse involvement with their infants postpartum. However, the authors noted that most mothers, even with depression and anxiety, were emotionally involved with their infants.

A prospective study of 88 women and their 7-month-old infants examined the link between prenatal anxiety disorder and mothers' caregiving sensitivity on infants' salivary cortisol (Grant et al., 2009). Maternal anxiety was assessed in the last 6 months of pregnancy. At 7 months, the infants' cortisol levels were measured 15, 25, and 40 minutes after exposure to the still-face mother procedure, a lab test where mothers do not respond to their babies' cues, which raises babies' cortisol levels (see p. 32). Mothers were classified as high- or low-sensitive based on analysis of video play sessions. Infants of low-sensitive mothers who had prenatal anxiety had a stronger stress response to the still-face procedure. In contrast, the infants of high-sensitive mothers had lower cortisol levels when they arrived at the laboratory compared to infants of less-sensitive mothers. Sensitive caregiving appeared to buffer elevated cortisol in novel and stressful situations.

A study of 2,888 mothers from the Upstate KIDS cohort (New York) found that mothers with prenatal depression were 36% to 62% more likely to have children with developmental delays (Putnick et al., 2022). There was a direct effect of prenatal depression on developmental delays, which may be due to in utero exposure to stress hormones. Postpartum depression and breastfeeding duration mediated this effect. Gestational age did not. Breastfeeding completely attenuated the effect of antenatal depression on fine motor development. The authors noted that breastfeeding initiation and duration may be a viable intervention to reduce developmental delays.

Emotional and Social Development

A study of mother–infant dyads up to age 9 months found that infants of depressed mothers had the poorest scores on measures of social engagement, maturity of regulatory behaviors, and negative emotionality (Feldman et al., 2009). Consistent with previous studies, infants of depressed mothers had the highest cortisol reactivity. The study compared 22 mother–infant dyads with maternal depression, 19 with maternal anxiety, and a group of matched controls. Maternal sensitivity moderated the effect of maternal depression on social engagement.

A study of mothers' PTSD showed similar results. In this study of 52 low-income, ethnic/minority mother–infant dyads found that they had experienced an average of 2.62 traumatic events, with 25% being exposed to 4 or more events (Enlow et al., 2011). Infants were assessed using the still-face paradigm at 6 months of age, and mothers completed a measure of infant temperament at 13 months. Consistent with previous studies, if mothers had high PTSD symptoms, their infants had more internalizing, externalizing, and dysregulation at 13 months. The authors concluded that maternal PTSD is related to infant difficulties with emotional regulation.

Mother–Infant Bonding

Depression can also make it more difficult for mothers to develop a warm, affectionate relationship with their babies, as a review of 67 studies found (Slomian et al., 2019). This was particularly an issue in the first 4 months, but depression impaired bonding at all time points. In this first year, depressed mothers were less attuned and showed less warmth, closeness, and sensitivity compared to non-depressed mothers. Not surprisingly, mothers reported more relationship difficulties and had more negative perceptions of their infants.

A study from Michigan examined the trajectory of mother–infant bonding over the first year in the context of maternal depression and history of childhood abuse (Muzik et al., 2013). They compared 97 women with a history of abuse to 53 non-abused women and assessed them at 6 weeks and at 4 and 6 months postpartum. All women increased in bonding over time, but postpartum depression or PTSD impaired bonding at each time point. What women thought about their babies also influenced their behavior. If they believed that they had not bonded with their babies, they had fewer positive parenting behaviors. The authors believed that early detection of depression and PTSD could prevent problematic parenting behaviors and disturbed mother–infant relationships.

A longitudinal study from London also examined the effects of postpartum depression over the first year (O'Higgins et al., 2013). There were 50 depressed mothers and 29 non-depressed mothers. Women who were depressed at 4 weeks did not bond well with their babies at all time points. The authors recommended early intervention.

A study of 180 women participating in a partial hospitalization program demonstrated that not all women with depression, or other psychiatric problems, have impaired bonding (Sockol et al., 2014). After controlling for demographic variables, they found that severe depression predicted impaired bonding and risk of abuse. Women having cesareans reported more rejection and pathological anger. Most of the women in the study had depression in the clinical range, but even compared to other depressed women, women with severe depression were at higher risk of bonding problems.

A German study compared 30 mothers with anxiety disorders and 48 without (Tietz et al., 2014). Mothers with anxiety disorders reported significantly less bonding with their babies than mothers without anxiety. However, some of this effect could also be explained by co-occurring depression.

Finally, a meta-analysis on 28 published and unpublished studies found that fathers' depression also affected parenting (Kitzman-Ulrich et al., 2010). Depressed fathers engaged in fewer positive, and more negative, parenting behaviors. The effect sizes found were comparable to studies on mothers. Positive behaviors included warm, sensitive, engaged, accepting, and supportive interactions. Negative behaviors included hostile, coercive, intrusive, restrictive, controlling, critical, and dysfunctional behaviors or interactions. The analysis revealed that mothers and fathers had comparable negative parenting behaviors, but the effect of depression on positive behaviors was larger for fathers than it is for mothers.

Infanticide

Infanticide is rare but always a tragedy. As I described in Chapter 1, depressed mothers can obsess over infant harm but do not actually do it. Unfortunately, some mothers do kill their babies, and it is important that we understand why so we can prevent it.

A study from Korea included 45 women who either killed or attempted to kill their infants (Kim et al., 2008). They collected data via chart review and examined whether depressive symptoms at admission predicted a later diagnosis of bipolar disorder. They found that while only 24% of the patients had a diagnosis of bipolar disorder at admission, 73% had this diagnosis at discharge. Among women admitted with a diagnosis of major depression, 65% were later reclassified based on the appearance of hypomanic or manic episodes. Healthcare providers should consider the diagnosis of bipolar disorder when examining filicidal depressive mothers. They also noted that patients with bipolar disorder should not be treated with antidepressants, which can trigger a manic episode. Indeed, 77% of their participants had been treated with antidepressants, with or without anti-psychotics.

Effects of Maternal Depression on Toddlers and Preschoolers

A review of 67 studies found significant consequences for children of depressed mothers (Slomian et al., 2019). Eleven studies found that mothers' depression was related to impaired cognitive development in children. However, three studies found no difference. Of 13 studies on language, 6 found that depression had a negative effect on children's language development, but 7 did not. Four of 5 studies found that children of depressed mothers had more fear and anxiety, impaired social development, and significant behavioral problems at age 2, including difficult temperament, more internalizing problems, and less mature self-regulation.

In a secondary analysis of data from the Healthy Steps National Evaluation with 3,412 mothers, depressed mothers at 2 to 4 months were less likely than non-depressed mothers to use electric outlet covers and safety latches, talk with their children, limit TV or video watching, follow daily routines, and be nurturing (McLearn et al., 2006)]. At 30 to 33 months, they were less likely to play with their children. Currently depressed mothers were more likely to slap their children's face or spank them with an object than non-depressed mothers.

Unfortunately, children who were premature may be more susceptible to the negative effects of maternal depression. In two studies, researchers measured children's cortisol levels after interacting with their mothers at 14 to 16 months (Bugental et al., 2008). Preterm infants had higher cortisol levels when interacting with their depressed mothers, but lower cortisol if their mothers were not depressed, compared to full-term infants. Premature infants were more sensitive to the emotional environment of their homes, including their mothers' depression.

A study of mother–child dyads (n = 838) assessed the impact of mothers' depression on children's adiposity at age 3 (Ertel et al., 2010). The mothers were predominantly White and affluent. Eight percent were depressed during pregnancy, and 7% were depressed postpartum. Mothers with prenatal depression had smaller babies at birth but had more central adiposity at age 3. Postpartum depression was also associated with higher child adiposity possibly because of the negative impact on breastfeeding, unhealthy maternal diet, and lower physical activity levels.

Effects on School-Aged Children

In a longitudinal study of 14,000 infants born in 2001, maternal depression increased the risk of childhood obesity at age 5 (Vericker, 2015). Low-income mothers were more likely to be depressed compared to affluent mothers, and 38% had recently been depressed. Children of depressed mothers ate fewer vegetables, drank less milk, drank sweetened beverages, and ate more sweet snacks compared to children of non-depressed mothers.

A prospective study of 65 mother–infant dyads found that mothers' high cortisol in early pregnancy increased right amygdala volume in girls, but not boys, at 7 years of age (Buss et al., 2012). This increased volume was related to girls' behavioral problems at age 7, as indicated by their score on the Child Behavior Checklist. There was no impact on the hippocampus for boys or girls.

Chronicity and severity of mothers' depression also influences child outcomes. A study of 3,332 mothers and children from Brazil identified psychiatric disorders in the children at age 6 (Matijasevich et al., 2015). The researchers identified five trajectories of maternal depression, ranging from low to high chronic. Thirteen percent of the children had a DSM-IV psychiatric disorder. The more severe their mothers' symptoms, the greater the probability of child psychiatric disorders, as well as internalizing and externalizing behaviors.

Ten-year-olds whose mothers had been depressed since their births (n = 17) were compared with children of non-depressed mothers (n = 21) on cortisol levels, hippocampal and amygdala volumes (Lupien et al., 2011). There were no differences in hippocampal volumes in children of depressed vs non-depressed mothers. However, children of depressed mothers had increased right and left amygdala volumes and increased levels of glucocorticoids compared to children of non-depressed mothers. Amygdala volume is a marker of biological sensitivity to quality of maternal care. Higher volume indicates distress.

Effects on Young Adults

Panic disorder was related to parenting behavior in a study of 86 Swiss mothers and their children, ages 13 to 23. Mothers with panic disorder were more verbally controlling, critical, and less sensitive during mother–child interactions than mothers without panic disorder (Lane et al., 2009). In structured-play situations, there were more conflicts between mother and child if the mothers had panic disorder. Parenting behaviors did not differ based on the children's anxiety levels. Parental overcontrol appears to undermine their children's self-efficacy.

A study of 150 pregnant women found that antenatal and postpartum depression predicted smoking in adolescent offspring (Hay et al., 2008). In this study, 31% of the mothers were depressed during pregnancy, and 22% were depressed at 3 months postpartum.

Mothers who were depressed at either time point were more likely to be depressed at subsequent assessment points. Perinatal depression predicted cumulative stress for families, which promoted adolescent disorders, including teen smoking.

A 20-year follow-up of children of depressed parents compared them with a matched group of children whose parents had no psychiatric illness. The adult children of depressed mothers and fathers had three times the rate of major depression, anxiety disorders, and substance use compared with children of non-depressed parents. In addition, children of depressed parents had higher rates of medical problems and premature mortality (Weissman et al., 2006).

A 22-year longitudinal Belgian study of postpartum depression found that the adult children of depressed mothers had a more reactive cortisol response to a perceived threat (a 5-minute speech followed by a 5-minute spoken mental-math test) compared to adult children of non-depressed mothers (Barry et al., 2015). There were 38 mother–child dyads in the depressed vs non-depressed groups.

The Interaction Styles of Depressed Mothers

Mothers' depression can lead to lasting and serious effects for their children. The next logical question to ask is why this occurs. Many studies have linked infant development difficulties to mothers' interaction style. Depression, anxiety, and PTSD can negatively impact these interactions. Most of this research has been done with depressed mothers.

In a study of 17 depressed and 19 non-depressed adolescent mothers, toddlers were observed in a cleanup task in order to observe parenting styles (Pelaez et al., 2008). The parenting styles were classified as (1) *Authoritative*, where mother provides firm control and set limits in a warm, respectful manner; (2) *Authoritarian*, where mother shows verbal or physical rejection, or control, or lacks positive encouragement; (3) *Permissive*, where mother provides positive verbal communication but sets no limits or provides no instructions; and (4) *Disengaged*, where mother is uninvolved, unresponsive, or avoidant and has flat affect. Depressed mothers were more likely to be classified as authoritarian or disengaged. Mothers' depression also appeared to affect their children's behaviors. The toddlers of depressed mothers spent less time following instructions, engaged in aggressive play for a greater percentage of time, and had less time on task than toddlers of non-depressed mothers.

Similarly, studies of depressed mothers have identified two basic interaction styles: avoidant and angry-intrusive (Field, 2010). Of these, the avoidant style is more common. Depressed mothers touch their infants less and are less physically affectionate. Their vocalizations also differ from those of non-depressed mothers. They use less repetition, have more negative affect, explain things less, and make fewer references to their infants' behavior. Depression reduces the synchrony between mothers and infants and has less infant-directed speech compared to that of non-depressed mothers.

The Still-Face Mother Studies

The Still-Face Mother Paradigm was developed by Dr. Edward Tronick to provide an analog, under laboratory conditions, of the effects of maternal depression. Tronick and colleagues asked mothers to mimic depressive symptoms when interacting with their 3-month-old babies by not responding to their cues for a short period of time (Grant et al., 2009; Liu et al., 2020). Mothers spoke in a monotone, had little or no facial affect, and seldom touched their infants. It only took about 3 minutes before the infants became distressed at the way their mothers were acting. The infants became wary and tried to engage their mothers in normal interactions. They continued to be wary even when mothers returned to their normal affect. It is highly stressful for infants when their mothers do not respond to them, and non-response elevates their cortisol (Buss et al., 2012).

Feeding Method Moderates the Interaction Style of Depressed Mothers

Surprisingly, very few researchers have examined whether feeding method influenced mothers' interaction style. I have only found one study that did (Jones et al., 2004). This study compared four groups of postpartum women: depressed women who were either breast- or bottle-feeding, and non-depressed women who were either breast- or bottle-feeding. The outcome was babies' electroencephalogram (EEG) patterns. In this study, babies of depressed/breastfeeding mothers had *normal* EEG patterns. In contrast, babies of depressed/non-breastfeeding women did not. In other words, *breastfeeding protected babies from the harmful effects of maternal depression.* The authors observed that depressed/breastfeeding mothers could not disengage from their babies because they had to engage to feed them. Compared to depressed/non-breastfeeding mothers, depressed/breastfeeding mothers touched, stroked, and made eye contact with their babies more than depressed/non-breastfeeding mothers because these behaviors are built into the breastfeeding relationship. I describe the research on breastfeeding and mothers' mental health more fully in Chapter 5.

Clinical Takeaways

- Depression causes more harm to mother and baby than people generally realize. These effects provide ample reason to take depression seriously and encourage mothers to seek treatment.
- In sharing information about infant harms, we must be careful to not communicate that mothers have somehow "ruined" their infants. Mothers fear this. In tragic cases, mothers with psychosis may mistakenly believe that their babies would be better off dead.
- Providers can, however, use this information to gently encourage mothers to seek help. Getting better also helps their babies.
- Breastfeeding protects babies whose mothers are depressed. Breastfeeding mothers touched, looked at, and spoke to the infants more than depressed/non-breastfeeding mothers.
- Non-breastfeeding mothers can be taught to interact with their infants and it lessens the harmful effects.

Section II

Underlying Mechanisms

5 Inflammation

The Underlying Mechanism for Postpartum Mental Illness

In 1998, Maes and Smith found that women with postpartum depression and anxiety had high levels of inflammation molecules in their plasma (Maes & Smith, 1998). At the time, the importance of this finding was not recognized, and inflammation was simply added to the growing list of risk factors. However, this finding turned out to be critical. We now know that inflammation is not a risk factor, per se, but the underlying physiologic mechanism that translates all risk factors into depressive symptoms. In other words, inflammation is not *a* risk factor; it's *the* risk factor, because it is the physiological mechanism that underlies all the others (Kendall-Tackett, 2007). Subsequent studies have shown that inflammation underlies anxiety, PTSD, bipolar disorder, and possibly even psychosis (Bergink et al., 2014; Gill et al., 2020). This chapter briefly describes the stress system and its opposing system: oxytocin.

KEY FINDINGS

- Inflammation is the underlying physiological mechanism in depression, anxiety, and PTSD. All effective treatments are also anti-inflammatory.
- The stress response has three main components: catecholamine response, hypothalamic-pituitary-adrenal (HPA) axis, and inflammatory-response system.
- The oxytocin system suppresses stress. Conversely, stress suppresses the oxytocin system.

Inflammation and Depression

Studies from the field of psychoneuroimmunology (PNI) have established inflammation as the process that "translates" risk factors into depression (i.e., our bodies respond to risk factors, such as pain or sleep deprivation, by increasing inflammation, which increases the risk for depression). Further, the relationship is bidirectional: inflammation increases depression (Duivis et al., 2015; Jaremka et al., 2013; Kiecolt-Glaser et al., 2015), and depression increases inflammation in response to stress. A study of 138 adults found that adults who were depressed had a stronger increase in inflammation response (IL-6) to a laboratory-induced stressor than those who were not depressed (Fagundes et al., 2013). IL-6 reliably predicted quality of life, morbidity, and many causes of mortality. A recent study also concluded that depression makes the inflammation response hyperreactive to current stressors (Worthen & Beurel, 2022).

DOI: 10.4324/9781003411246-7

In this edition, I separate underlying mechanisms from risk factors to emphasize their relative importance. More than 20 years ago, Maes (2001) recognized inflammation as the underlying mechanism in depression.

The discovery that psychological stress can induce the production of proinflammatory cytokines has important implications for human psychopathology and, in particular, for the aetiology of major depression. Psychological stressors, such as negative life events, are emphasized in the aetiology of depression. Thus, psychosocial and environmental stressors play a role as direct precipitants of major depression. or they function as vulnerability factors which predispose humans to develop major depression. *Major depression is accompanied by activation of the inflammatory response system (IRS) with, among other things, an increased production of proinflammatory cytokines, such as IL-1β, IL-6, TNF-α, and an acute-phase response.*

(Maes, 2001, p. 193, emphasis added)

In other words, inflammation is the key to understanding everything. It explains the link between physical and psychological stress and depression, explains the role of breastfeeding in mothers' mental health, helps us understand why depression and anxiety increase the risk of heart disease and diabetes, and finally, it helps us understand why all effective treatments for depression are anti-inflammatory.

The Anti-Stress Effect

Fortunately, our bodies offer a counterresponse to chronic stress. The oxytocin system promotes physical and mental health and works in opposition to the stress system. These systems mutually suppress each other. When one system is upregulated, the other is suppressed (Uvnas-Moberg, 2015). It is like a light switch: when the light is on, light suppresses the darkness. Conversely, off suppresses light. Both systems are controlled by a section of the hypothalamus called the paraventricular nucleus (PVN) (Uvnas-Moberg et al., 2020). The key to improving mothers' mental health is activating the oxytocin system, which suppresses the stress system and the inflammatory response.

The oxytocin vs stress response also helps us understand why studies sometimes have contradictory results. Findings can vary depending on which system is upregulated. One example is breastfeeding's impact on mothers' mental health. If breastfeeding is going well (i.e., oxytocin is upregulated), it lowers the risk of depression and other mental health conditions. In contrast, if mothers are in pain or are worried about their milk supply (i.e., stress is upregulated), mothers' risk of depression increases.

This chapter describes both the stress and oxytocin systems. The subsequent chapter describes the role of breastfeeding as part of the physiological mechanism that activates either the stress or oxytocin systems.

The Stress System

Stress is a necessary part of life. We could not get out of bed without the stress response and would find it difficult to make it through the day. Our stress response is also adaptive;

it protects us from danger and keeps us alive. When the stress system is working the way that it should, it should turn on when it is needed and then turn off when it is not. Problems arise when stress becomes chronic, and the stress response is activated long-term. The three main components of the stress system are as follows.

Catecholamine Response

The catecholamine response, or fight-or-flight response, is the one most people identify as the "stress response." As the name implies, it gives you the strength to run away or fight your way through it. In response to threat or danger, we release three neurotransmitters: epinephrine (adrenaline), norepinephrine, and dopamine. The catecholamine response is instant and activated in response to physical or psychological threat.

Hypothalamic-Pituitary-Adrenal (HPA) Axis

Another component of the stress system is the HPA axis. It is a cascade response involving three structures. The hypothalamus releases a stress hormone called corticotrophin releasing hormone (CRH), which causes the pituitary to release adrenocorticotropin hormone (ACTH), which causes the cortex of the adrenal glands to release cortisol.

The regulation of the HPA axis changes markedly during pregnancy. The placenta also produces CRH, and not solely the hypothalamus, as it does when women are not pregnant. Cortisol stimulates CRH in the placenta rather than downregulating it, as it does when the hypothalamus produces it. One study found that elevated CRH in pregnancy strongly predicted postpartum depression (Yim et al., 2009). Serum samples from 100 pregnant women were assayed for CRH, ACTH, and cortisol five times during pregnancy. Depression was assessed four times prenatally and once postpartum. Elevated CRH at 25 weeks' gestation predicted postpartum depression, but not at the other time points.

A study of 284 mothers from Sweden found high prenatal cortisol increased the risk of depression by 4 times (Illiadis et al., 2015). Researchers examined evening cortisol levels and assessed mothers at 18 and 36 weeks' gestation and 6 weeks postpartum. They controlled for history of depression, smoking, partner support, breastfeeding, stressful life events, and sleep problems.

Inflammatory Response System

Inflammation is the final part of the stress response. In response to threat or danger, our bodies release inflammation molecules called proinflammatory (increases inflammation) cytokines (Corwin & Pajer, 2008; Kendall-Tackett, 2007). Researchers assess systemic inflammation by measuring serum levels of proinflammatory cytokines. The proinflammatory cytokines identified most often in depression research are interleukin-1β (IL-1β), interleukin-6 (IL-6), and tumor necrosis factor-α (TNF-α). Researchers sometimes use another measure of inflammation, called C-reactive protein (CRP). A logical question to ask is why our bodies increase inflammation in response to threat. The answer lies in their function. Inflammation molecules fight infection and heal wounds. If your body believes that it is in danger, it will increase inflammation in case you are wounded.

When Stress is Chronic

Maes and Smith (1998) described several plausible explanations for why inflammation increases depression risk. First, when inflammation levels are high, people experience classic symptoms of depression, such as fatigue, lethargy, and social withdrawal. Researchers demonstrated that inflammation has a causal role in depression when using inflammatory cytokines as chemotherapy for conditions such as cancer or hepatitis. When patients are treated with cytokines, depression increases in a predictable and dose–response way: the greater the dosage of cytokines, the more depressed the patients. When the dose is tapered, depression drops (Baumeister et al., 2016; Kiecolt-Glaser et al., 2015). Second, inflammation activates the hypothalamic-pituitary-adrenal (HPA) axis, dysregulating levels of cortisol. Cortisol, as an endogenous corticosteroid, generally keeps inflammation in check. However, depression dysregulates cortisol, which then fails to restrain the inflammatory response (Dhabhar & McEwen, 2001). Finally, inflammation decreases serotonin by lowering levels of its precursor, tryptophan. Treating both inflammation and depression together improves outcomes (Chen & Lacey, 2018; Kiecolt-Glaser et al., 2015).

A review by Bergink et al. (2014) found that inflammation was likely the underlying cause of bipolar disorder, schizophrenia, and postpartum psychosis. They also noted high co-occurrence of autoimmune disorders in people with psychosis, which suggests that autoimmunity and psychosis are two manifestations of the same underlying processes.

Why Inflammation is Particularly Relevant to Depression in New Mothers

Pregnant and postpartum women are particularly vulnerable to the effects of inflammation because it normally increases during the last trimester of pregnancy—a time when they are also at highest risk for depression (Kendall-Tackett, 2007). Indeed, elevated cytokines in the last trimester match the pattern of perinatal depression more accurately than the pattern of other biological markers, such as the rise and fall of reproductive hormones (Corwin et al., 2015).

Inflammation is also high right after giving birth (Corwin et al., 2015). One study found that postpartum women are generally higher in the cytokines IL-6, IL-6R, and IL-IRA than before delivery (Maes et al., 2000). Corwin and Johnston's (2008) sample included 38 women in the first 24 hours after delivery. High IL-1β on day 14 was associated with depression on day 28. The authors recommended addressing inflammation directly with anti-inflammatory interventions, including using NSAIDS, early diagnosis and treatment of subclinical infections, and careful wound care, so that these interventions might reduce the development of postpartum depression.

A study from Greece recruited 56 pregnant women and recorded a detailed medical and obstetric history (Boufidou et al., 2009). The researchers measured postpartum blues at 1 and 4 days postpartum and depression at 1 and 6 weeks. They measured blood and cerebrospinal fluid (CSF) and found that women with depressive symptoms at day 4 and week 6 had elevated TNF-α and IL-6 in their blood and CSF. CSF is a more sensitive measure of central nervous system activity than blood.

Corwin and colleagues (2015) tested whether the bidirectional interaction between the inflammatory response system and HPA axis increased women's risk of postpartum depression in a sample of 152 women. They found that family history of depression, day 14 cortisol AUC (area under the curve), and day 14 IL-8/IL-10 ratio predicted depressive symptoms. They concluded that cytokines and the HPA axis integrate to influence postpartum mood.

One recent study proceeded under the assumption that inflammation caused postpartum depression and examined whether mothers' use of ibuprofen prevented it (Kapulsky et al., 2021). The sample was prospective and included 54 women who were assessed at 3 and 6 weeks postpartum. Ibuprofen lowered the risk of depression, but only for the mothers not currently taking psychotropic medications. Acetaminophen, which is not anti-inflammatory, did not lower risk.

Oxytocin: The Anti-Stress System

The oxytocin and stress systems mutually oppose each other; when oxytocin is upregulated, it suppresses the stress response. Oxytocin functions as a neurotransmitter in the brain and is a hormone in the body. It is highly anti-inflammatory and has been used to treat inflammatory conditions such as sepsis (Mehdi et al., 2022), cardiovascular disease (Jankowski et al., 2020), and even to counter the hyperinflammation associated with COVID-19, which was considered a better option than glucocorticoids (Buemann et al., 2021). Even on a cellular level, activation of the oxytocin receptors reduced IL-6 (Szeto et al., 2017).

During labor, oxytocin contracts the uterus and is released when babies' heads press on their mothers' cervixes. It also facilitates mother–infant attachment and helps mothers cope with monotony and the stresses of new motherhood (Uvnas-Moberg, 2015). Oxytocin causes milk ejection during breastfeeding. When mothers are frightened or in extreme pain, stress is activated and oxytocin is suppressed, which causes labor to stall (Uvnas-Moberg, 2015). The same is true for early breastfeeding. Stress, cold, strangers in the room, or pain can delay when milk "comes in" (lactogenesis II) by several days, because these stressors suppress oxytocin and prolactin, the hormone that makes milk.

Synthetic oxytocin, used to induce and augment labor, is not the same as endogenous oxytocin. If used during labor, synthetic oxytocin increased the risk for postpartum depression and anxiety in a large population study (Kroll-Desrosiers et al., 2017). Strangely, the authors predicted that synthetic oxytocin would decrease mothers' risk of depression and anxiety and were surprised when it did not. I was surprised that they were surprised. Their finding is exactly what I would have expected. Synthetic oxytocin makes labor very painful, which would activate the stress system. In addition, it is peripheral (stays in the body) and does not cross the blood-brain barrier so would have no impact on mothers' mental health. If a woman's labor was more painful, I would expect exactly what they found: more depression and anxiety.

Throughout the lifespan, high oxytocin makes you like other people and want to be around them. You trust them. Oxytocin makes life enjoyable and is the opposite of the stress response. Oxytocin is typically associated with love, attachment, and closeness (Uvnas-Moberg, 2013). It is also released during orgasm.

Breastfeeding affects mental health because it upregulates oxytocin and suppresses the stress response (Kendall-Tackett, 2007). Skin-to-skin contact also increases oxytocin (Handlin et al., 2009). Social support also increases oxytocin, and a recent meta-analysis found that it is also anti-inflammatory (Uchino et al., 2018). I describe this effect in more detail in the next chapter.

Clinical Takeaways

- Inflammation is the underlying physiological process for mental health disorders.
- Oxytocin suppresses the stress system and lowers risk for depression and other mental health disorders.
- Treatments that suppress inflammation and increase oxytocin will be the most effective.

6 Breastfeeding
Nature's Method to Protect Mothers' Mental Health

Breastfeeding[1] is often presented as merely a "feeding choice," where mothers are trying to give their babies a "slightly better" product. Why cause mothers the extra stress? To frame breastfeeding like this misses a critical point. Breastfeeding is far more than providing milk for a baby. Breastfeeding is a sophisticated and integrated system that protects mothers and babies and helps them both navigate postpartum stresses. Yes, breastfeeding can be stressful in the beginning, but that stress indicts the maternity systems that fail to provide proper support and is not a reason to encourage mothers to avoid it.

I have included breastfeeding in this section on mechanisms because of its impact on the stress system. In the previous chapter, I described oxytocin's effect on the stress system, which decreases mothers' risk of depression. Breastfeeding mothers can still get depressed, but it lowers their risk. If they are depressed, breastfeeding lessens their symptoms (Figueiredo et al., 2021).

KEY FINDINGS

- Women who are exclusively breastfeeding have lower rates of depression.
- Exclusive breastfeeding downregulates the stress response by upregulating oxytocin.
- Mothers who want to breastfeed and stop prematurely are at even higher risk for depression than mothers who never start.

Breastfeeding Downregulates the Stress Response

Maureen Gröer and colleagues (2002) were the first to identify breastfeeding's important role in downregulating the stress response. She noted that breastfeeding confers a survival advantage that protects the mother and directs her toward milk production, conservation of energy, and nurturing behaviors (Groer et al., 2002). Hormones related to lactation, such as oxytocin and prolactin, have both antidepressant and anxiolytic effects (Mezzacappa & Endicott, 2007).

Figueiredo et al. (2013) described possible mechanisms by which breastfeeding might protect maternal mental health:

1. By promoting hormonal processes that suppress cortisol
2. By regulating sleep for mother and child
3. By increasing the mother's self-efficacy and emotional connection with her baby
4. By reducing difficulties related to child temperament
5. By promoting better mother–infant interaction (Figueiredo et al., 2013)

DOI: 10.4324/9781003411246-8

A recent study examined the impact of breastfeeding on allostatic load in a US population sample (Hsiao & Sibeko, 2021). *Allostatic load* is a composite of stress biomarkers and is a better predictor of health effects than individual markers. The authors examined 10 waves of NHANES[2] data from 1999 to 2018 (*n* = 1,302) controlling for maternal age, race and ethnicity, education, poverty level, and survey wave. Breastfeeding significantly lowered allostatic load. They concluded that oxytocin downregulated the stress response and influenced multiple body systems, showing benefits beyond a single biomarker.

> This downregulation of stress is particularly important during the postpartum period when mothers are susceptible to higher levels of stress and inflammation in the third trimester of pregnancy, and the need to recover from childbirth stress, pain, trauma, and sleep disturbances that are commonplace in the postpartum period.
>
> (p. 7)

A recent review of 29 articles on breastfeeding and oxytocin had similar findings (Uvnas-Moberg et al., 2020). Oxytocin is released in pulses during the first 10 to 20 minutes of suckling. Breastfeeding-induced oxytocin release increased levels of prolactin, the hormone necessary for milk production. Oxytocin directly lowers ACTH and cortisol and decreases activation of the sympathetic nervous system. Prolactin is less susceptible to stress but can be affected indirectly via oxytocin. Oxytocin also lowers anxiety and aggression and increases sensitivity to others.

Another systematic review of 12 articles found an inverse relationship between endogenous oxytocin and depression in 8 studies: when oxytocin was high, depressive symptoms were low (Thul et al., 2020). Interestingly, they controlled for breastfeeding, which they considered a confounder. Not surprisingly, because it does not cross the blood-brain barrier, intravenous oxytocin did not lower risk of depression.

A recent study from Nepal (*n* = 162) compared the stress levels of exclusively breastfeeding (*n* = 81) and non-breastfeeding mothers (*n* = 81) (Kharel et al., 2020). Perceived stress and systolic blood pressure were significantly higher in the non-breastfeeding mothers than the breastfeeding mothers. They noted that oxytocin and prolactin have antidepressant, anti-anxiolytic, and anti-stress effects.

Prolactin, the hormone that makes milk, was also hypothesized to increase mothers' sensitivity to their infants (Hahn-Holbrook et al., 2021). In a sample of 28 infants, half were assigned to breastfeeding and half bottle-fed with their expressed milk. Researchers measured prolactin 40 minutes after each feeding session and then recorded mothers free-playing with their infants. Mothers who fed at the breast were more sensitive to infant cues than mothers who bottle-fed their breastmilk. Prolactin levels did not differ between the groups, but prolactin level was positively associated with sensitivity. The authors concluded that feeding directly at the breast increased maternal sensitivity, likely due to oxytocin.

A study of 43 breastfeeding women examined the effects of baby at the breast vs holding their babies without breastfeeding on the HPA axis. Babies suckling at the breast significantly decreased ACTH, plasma cortisol, and salivary free cortisol (Heinrichs et al., 2001). Breastfeeding and holding the infant significantly decreased anxiety, but mood and calmness improved only after the baby was at the breast. When deliberately stressed in the lab, breastfeeding suppressed the HPA axis and suppressed the stress response short-term. The researchers argued that this short-term suppression provided several evolutionary and biological advantages: it isolated the mother from distracting stimuli, facilitated her immune response, protected the baby from high cortisol in the milk, and prevented stress-related inhibition of lactation.

A study of 63 primiparous mothers at 2 days postpartum had similar findings (Handlin et al., 2009). Breastfeeding lowered ACTH and cortisol, and skin-to-skin contact contributed to these effects. Suckling decreased ACTH, and skin-to-skin contact decreased cortisol. Oxytocin also reduced ACTH and cortisol during breastfeeding.

Population studies also find lower rates of depression in breastfeeding vs non-breastfeeding women. In a sample of 209 low-income women from Oklahoma, formula feeding doubled the risk of depression (McCoy et al., 2006). Thirty-nine percent of this sample was depressed. A study from Croatia had similar findings (Miksic et al., 2020). Two hundred and nine women were assessed during pregnancy, immediately postpartum, and at 3 months. Mothers who did not breastfeed were more depressed than mothers who did. Anxiety was also higher when mothers breastfed for a shorter time.

US PRAMS[3] data from 31 sites (n = 32,659) showed that women with the highest rate of depression were those who breastfed for less than 8 weeks (15.6%) compared to those who never breastfed (14%) and those who breastfed more than 8 weeks (11.8%) (Bauman et al., 2020). A study of 1,037 women from Crete also found that breastfeeding for less than 8 weeks increased the risk for depression (Koutra et al., 2018). These findings suggest that mothers who initiate breastfeeding and stop early are at even higher risk for depression than those who never start. Breastfeeding support in the early weeks also protects women's mental health.

In Pakistan, 17% of a sample of 434 new mothers were depressed (Shah & Lonegan, 2017). Mothers who were mixed feeding were 2.3 times more likely to be depressed than those who were exclusively breastfeeding. Other risk factors were lack of husband and family support, which increased the risk by 6 times, and a 90% increased risk if their youngest child was a girl.

Long-Term Health Effects for Breastfeeding Mothers

Breastfeeding's downregulation of the stress response also has long-term effects on women's risk of cardiovascular disease (Schwartz et al., 2009). This study included 139,681 postmenopausal women (mean age = 63 years). The researchers found that women with a lifetime history of breastfeeding for more than 12 months were less likely to have hypertension, diabetes, hyperlipidemia, or cardiovascular disease than women who never breastfed. This was a dose–response relationship: the longer women lactated, the lower their cardiovascular risk. The authors noted that lactation improves glucose tolerance, lipid metabolism, and C-reactive protein.

Breastfeeding may also influence infants' emotional development. In a study of 28 8-month-olds, researchers compared babies who were low exclusive breastfeeding (12 to 152 days) and high exclusive breastfeeding (167 to 252 days) on neural processing of images of happiness or fear (Krol et al., 2015). Babies who were high exclusive breastfeeding paid more attention to happy stimuli, and those who were low exclusive breastfeeding paid more attention to fear stimuli. The authors speculated that exclusive breastfeeding affects central oxytocin levels in infants, which biases them toward either positive or negative information.

Prospective Studies of Depression and Breastfeeding

Some people have asked me how I know *breastfeeding* lowers the risk of depression and not some other factor. Since depressed mothers are less likely to breastfeed, they have already self-selected into a non-breastfeeding group in studies. That is true, and it is an issue than can be addressed by study design. With a typical survey, we cannot tell whether breastfeeding protects mothers' mental health, but we can with a prospective study.

Prospective studies are gold standard for determining whether breastfeeding influences mental health. With this design, researchers assess depression in both groups at the beginning of the study to make sure that each group only included mothers who were not depressed. By time 2, if mothers in the bottle-feeding group are more depressed, researchers can conclude that feeding method influenced mothers' mental health.

These studies reveal that only *exclusive* breastfeeding protects mental health. Mixed feeding, which provides many benefits for both mother and baby, does not appear to downregulate the stress response enough to protect mothers from depression. These results are consistent with our and Doheim et al.'s survey findings (Dorheim et al., 2009a; Kendall-Tackett et al., 2011; Kendall-Tackett, 2013, #2602). These studies suggest that exclusive breastfeeding changes physiology in a way that mixed feeding does not.

A prospective study of 2,072 women from Malaysia also examined the relationship between exclusive breastfeeding and depression at 1 and 3 months postpartum (Yusuff et al., 2016). Exclusively breastfeeding mothers had significantly lower depression scores at both time points than mothers who never breastfed or who were not exclusively breastfeeding. This relationship remained significant even after controlling for covariates.

A prospective study of 205 pregnant women found that women who breastfed more frequently at 3 months postpartum had significantly lower depressive symptoms by 24 months (Hahn-Holbrook et al., 2013). Depression was measured at 5 points during pregnancy, and 4 times up to 24 months. Mothers who breastfed 9 times a day or more were significantly less depressed than mothers who breastfed less than 4 times a day, even after controlling for age, income, education, social support, and employment status.

A Spanish study of 711 breastfeeding mothers found that exclusive breastfeeding was associated with lower stress at 1 month postpartum than mixed feeding (Gila-Diaz et al., 2020). At 3 months, mothers who were mixed feeding were more stressed and depressed than those who were exclusively breastfeeding. In this study, the researchers defined exclusive breastfeeding differently than other studies: exclusive feeding of the mothers' own milk, but not necessarily at the breast. Yet they found the same effect.

A prospective study of 334 mothers from Portugal included 70 mothers who were depressed during their pregnancies and 197 mothers who were not depressed (Figueiredo et al., 2021). They assessed mothers in their 3rd trimester and at 3 to 6 months postpartum. If women were depressed during pregnancy, exclusive breastfeeding lessened symptoms and lowered rates of depression between 3 and 6 months postpartum. Exclusive breastfeeding did not lower the risk of depression for the non-depressed women.

Other researchers examined IL-6 and cortisol in 119 women were recruited during pregnancy and followed through 6 months postpartum (Ahn & Corwin, 2015). They were assessed during the third trimester, on days 7 and 14 postpartum, and at 1–3, and 6 months. The rates of breastfeeding "most of the time" were 92% at day 7, and 71% at 6 months—well over US national averages. Depression or perceived stress did not differ for breastfeeding vs bottle-feeding mothers at 6 months. However, salivary cortisol levels at 8:00 a.m. and 8:30 a.m. were higher (indicating that the HPA axis was functioning well), and IL-6 was lower, for the mothers predominantly breastfeeding at 6 months. One factor that may have influenced their findings was their measure of breastfeeding. Physiologically, "predominant breastfeeding" may not be the same as *exclusive breastfeeding*. In our previous study, there was no difference between mixed-feeding and formula-feeding mothers on measures of depression, anxiety, or sleep (Kendall-Tackett et al., 2011). But Ahn and Corwin's findings suggest that even when not exclusively breastfeeding, inflammation and cortisol were still positively affected.

Mothers' Intention to Breastfeed

Mothers' breastfeeding goals are important. If mothers plan to breastfeed and cannot, then lack of breastfeeding becomes a risk factor for depression. It is important to address this because healthcare providers often believe that they are helping when they encourage depressed mothers to not start or to wean. For mothers who want to quit, that can be helpful. But a surprising number want to continue, and people try to talk them out of it. Speaking about nurses, McCarter-Spaulding and Horowitz noted the following:

> Nurses caring for women who are at-risk, or struggling with PPD, also may feel that breastfeeding is perhaps an unnecessary burden that should be discontinued.
>
> Although nurses might expect that mothers with depression may not want to continue, or may not be able to maintain breastfeeding, such assumptions may not be accurate
>
> (McCarter-Spaulding & Horowitz, 2007, p. 10)

I have also spoken with hundreds of mothers who had been diagnosed with postpartum depression and told to wean. Many said, "But this is the only thing that is going well." Telling these mothers to wean does not help and may keep them from seeking treatment. Actress Brooke Shields eloquently described her experience.

> Both my mother-in-law and my mother suggested that I stop breastfeeding to give myself a break. . . . [N]obody understood that breastfeeding was my only real connection to the baby. If I were to eliminate that, I might have no hope of coming through this nightmare. I was hanging on to breastfeeding as my lifeline. It was the only thing that made me unique in terms of caring for her. . . . Without it, she might be lost to me forever.
>
> Brooke Shields (Shields, 2005, pp. 80–81)

Recent studies on mothers' intention to breastfeed also support these personal observations. The Avon Longitudinal Study of Parents and Children (ALSPAC) found that intention to breastfeed was an important predictor of postpartum depression (Borra et al., 2015). Mothers who were not depressed during pregnancy had the lowest risk of depression if they planned to breastfeed their babies and were able to do it. *Mothers who planned to breastfeed but could not were at highest risk.* The authors recommended that mothers receive skilled breastfeeding support so that they could meet their goals. Mothers who could not breastfeed need compassionate care.

Mothers from the Infant Feeding Practices Study II (*n* = 1,501) were included if they intended to exclusively breastfeed (Gregory et al., 2015). Thirty-nine percent exclusively breastfed, and 23% had depressive symptoms. Mothers who met their prenatal goals had fewer depressive symptoms than mothers who did not, if they were middle- or upper-income. This was not true for the lower-income mothers.

Mental Health and Breastfeeding Cessation

Breastfeeding and mental health intersect in some interesting ways: breastfeeding protects mothers' mental health, but mothers with depression, anxiety, or PTSD are less likely to start or exclusively breastfeed and more likely to stop early. Early cessation and lack of exclusive breastfeeding both increase mothers' risk for depression. Obviously, timely breastfeeding support can help and should be part of mental healthcare.

Depression

A US nationally representative sample of 1,271 mothers, who were part of the Infant Feeding Practices Study II cited earlier, found that women with depressive symptoms breastfed, and exclusively breastfed, for a shorter time than mothers who were not depressed (Bascom & Napolitano, 2016). Sore nipples were also more common in the depressed mothers. Sixty-nine percent of the total sample stopped breastfeeding before 6 months, with "too many household duties" cited as the most common reason, which suggests an overall lack of support.

Hahn-Holbrook et al. (2013) found that mothers with prenatal depression were less likely to breastfeed and weaned on average of 2.3 months earlier than non-depressed mothers. A study of 873 families from Finland found an indirect relationship between prenatal depression and non-exclusive breastfeeding; prenatal depression increased the risk of postpartum depression, which led to non-exclusive breastfeeding (Ahlqvist-Bjorkroth et al., 2016).

A study of 229 women from Chile found that women with prenatal depression or anxiety, or who were currently depressed and anxious, were more likely to mixed- or formula-feed at 3 months (Coo et al., 2020). However, if women were exclusively breastfeeding at 3 months, they were more likely to continue to 6 months. American Latinas (*n* = 34) who were depressed during pregnancy or postpartum, or who were anxious postpartum, were more likely to stop breastfeeding by 8 weeks than the non-depressed women (Lara-Cinisomo et al., 2017). Women who were depressed and stopped breastfeeding had lower oxytocin than non-depressed women. Did low oxytocin (because of depression) make them stop or did oxytocin drop when they stopped? Very interesting question for a future study.

A prospective study of first-time Australian mothers also found depression led to breastfeeding cessation: 49% of mothers depressed at 3 months postpartum were breastfeeding at 6 months compared to 61% of non-depressed mothers (Woolhouse et al., 2016). Groër and Morgan (2007) found that women depressed at 4 to 6 weeks postpartum were significantly less likely to breastfeed, had lower serum prolactin levels, and had more life stress and anxiety in their sample of 200 women.

Researchers in Southeast Brazil studied 168 new mothers and found that depressive symptoms and traumatic deliveries both predicted lack of exclusive breastfeeding at 2 months (Machado et al., 2014). A study of 2,589 mother–infant pairs in Northeast Brazil also found that depressed mothers, or those with late prenatal care, were less likely to exclusively breastfeed (Silva et al., 2017).

A qualitative study from Ghana included three focus groups: new mothers, fathers, and grandmothers. All acknowledged the impact of depression on breastfeeding (Scorza et al., 2015). Study participants described depression as "thinking too much." One grandmother said, "[S]he thinks too much; the child doesn't get breast milk to suck because breast milk is not available." Grandmothers reported that babies refuse to feed if "a woman has not happiness[;] her baby can see that her mother is sad by looking at the mother's face, in which case the baby would not breastfeed." Fathers also noted that depressed women become withdrawn and do not eat. If they do not eat well, they cannot produce enough milk for breastfeeding.

One hundred twenty-two depressed women described their breastfeeding experiences (McCarter-Spaulding & Horowitz, 2007). Depression was most severe at 4 to 6 weeks and dropped off after that. By 14 to 18 weeks postpartum, 78% were no longer depressed. All were encouraged to seek treatment for depression, but only 11% to 12% had gone to psychotherapy, and 3% to 6% used medications. At 14 to 18 weeks, 33% were mixed-feeding and 45% were exclusively formula-feeding. Depression had the largest impact on exclusive breastfeeding (McCarter-Spaulding & Horowitz, 2007).

Nipple Pain, Depression, and Breastfeeding Cessation

Pain is related to both depression and breastfeeding cessation. It tells our bodies that something is wrong, which negates breastfeeding's protection. In my opinion, it is unconscionable when lactation providers tell mothers, "That should get better in a bit. Just keep going." (I know that some providers say this, because those mothers eventually come to me.)

Mental health practitioners aid and abet this harmful response because they may assume that pain is a "normal" part of breastfeeding, probably because so many mothers they see have it. Studies have found that 50% of women had nipple pain at 5 weeks postpartum (McGovern et al., 2006) and 52% of mothers had cracked or sore nipples (Ansara et al., 2005). I am outraged that these mothers suffered for so long. The system, and specific providers, clearly failed them. Good breastfeeding support can eliminate nipple pain, often quickly. To mental health practitioners, I would say this: *while nipple pain is common, **it is not normal**, and it should be addressed immediately with skilled lactation care. If one provider cannot help, find someone else. This is critical for mothers' mental health*.

Pain tells our bodies that we are under attack, which triggers an inflammatory response and increases the risk for depression. Proinflammatory cytokines (especially IL-1) are stimulated by substance P, the neuropeptide associated with pain. High substance P increases proinflammatory cytokines, which increase prostaglandin synthesis, which increases pain and starts a very harmful downward cycle.

A study of 2,586 women in the US found that breastfeeding pain at Day 1, Week 1, or Week 2 increased depression at 2 months (Watkins et al., 2011). Severe pain doubled the odds of postpartum depression, and depressed women were significantly less likely to still be breastfeeding at 2 months. *However, if they received breastfeeding help, it protected their mental health even if they had moderate or severe pain.* This was likely caused by social support's upregulation of oxytocin, which downregulated the stress response.

In a study of 229 postpartum women from Melbourne, Australia, researchers found that breastfeeding problems, with or without concurrent health problems, increased the risk of postpartum depression at 8 weeks (Cooklin et al., 2018). "High burden" breast-feeding problems included 2 or more of the following: nipple pain, frequent expressing, over- or undersupply. "High burden" physical health problems included 2 or more of the following: cesarean or perineal pain, back pain, constipation, or hemorrhoids, and urinary or bowel incontinence.

Anxiety

Anxiety can also lead to premature weaning. A systematic review of 33 studies found that women with postpartum anxiety were less likely to initiate breastfeeding and more likely to supplement in the hospital than women without anxiety (Fallon et al., 2016). Anxiety also reduced breastfeeding self-efficacy, which predicted breastfeeding duration. Data from a longitudinal pregnancy cohort study ($n = 412$) revealed that every unit of pregnancy-specific anxiety decreased exclusive breastfeeding by 5% to 6% at 6 to 8 weeks (Horsely et al., 2019).

Japanese researchers, in a study of 2,020 new mothers, found that mothers with anxiety were less likely to exclusively breastfeed (Fukui et al., 2021). Depression did not have this effect, and type of breastfeeding did not significantly affect depression in the early postpartum period. Feeding method was not related to mother–infant bonding, but mothers who were higher in mother–infant bonding were more likely to exclusively breastfeed at 6 months.

Posttraumatic Stress Disorder

Posttraumatic stress disorder can also influence breastfeeding. Traumatic childbirth and posttraumatic stress disorder (PTSD) lowered breastfeeding self-efficacy at 3 months postpartum in a prospective longitudinal study of 102 Turkish women (Turkmen et al., 2020). In a sample of 1,480 women from the Akershus Birth Cohort study, women with postpartum PTSD were 6 times less likely to initiate breastfeeding and continue to 12 months compared to women without postpartum PTSD (Garthus-Niegel et al., 2018). The authors emphasized the importance of screening new mothers for PTSD. A systematic review of 26 samples found that mothers with PTSD were less likely to breastfeed than mothers without PTSD, and that PTSD had a negative impact on mother–infant interaction (Cook et al., 2018).

Mothers' Experiences of Breastfeeding after Sexual Abuse

Sexual abuse is a common form of trauma, and the subjective experiences of abuse survivors who breastfeed vary quite a bit. Mothers' feelings about breastfeeding can overlap with their trauma experiences. Following are two accounts of women's experiences. First, Beth Dubois (2003) describes how she was nervous about breastfeeding, and wondered if it was possible, but ultimately found it healing and empowering.

> As the time of my son's birth approached, my worries about breastfeeding came into sharp focus. . . . I knew I wanted to breastfeed. I had been sexually abused when I was a child, however, and I was concerned. I worried that . . . the constant physical closeness breastfeeding would require . . . might trigger memories of the

abuse. I was especially distraught because I believed that I would be failing my child and myself if I were not able to breastfeed. . . .

. . . I now see that not only has breastfeeding been possible for me, a survivor of childhood sexual abuse, it has been immensely healing. My desire to have a fulfilling breastfeeding relationship forced me to face emotional territory I would probably have otherwise avoided. One wound left by the abuse is an underlying sense of "I can't do it. It's not even worth trying." Birthing and breastfeeding Theodore has helped to replace this with a very real sense of capability and confidence. Also, the heightened sensitivity to both me and my son, which I gained through our breastfeeding relationship, serves us in other ways, especially now that Theodore is in the "terrific twos."

(pp. 50–51)

Unfortunately, some survivors find breastfeeding so difficult that they need to stop. Beck (2009) presented the story of a woman who survived childhood sexual abuse and rape as an adult. During her birth, she dissociated and had a flashback to her abuse experience.

A haze of hospital labor room, nakedness, vulnerability, pain. Silence, stretching, breathing, pain terror, and then I found myself 7 years old again, and sitting outside my parents' house in the car of a family acquaintance, being digitally raped. . . . [M]y birth experience did not look traumatic at all—because the trauma physically took place 23 years before and only in my mind, not the labor room.

(Beck, 2009, pp. e4–e5)

After birth, her milk supply was very low, possibly due to her traumatic birth or her preeclampsia. Her inability to breastfeed compounded her feelings of shame and inadequacy. She felt numb postpartum and could not connect with her baby, husband, or life.

Of course, I couldn't tell anyone what was really going on in my head when I tried to breastfeed. When I placed my baby to the breast, I experienced panic attacks, spaced out, and dissociated. . . . I hated the physical feeling of breastfeeding. . . . Whenever I put her to breast, I wanted to scream and vomit at the same time. . . . The very act of breastfeeding, which was sustaining my baby, was forcing me to relive the abuse. I resented her for needing to breastfeed. . . . I did actually experience some relief when I expressed, rather than breastfeeding directly; however, my supply was poor. . . . [W]hen I gave myself permission to give up on breastfeeding, things started to look up. I slowly started to feel a sense of connection with my baby, and with my life, and I even began to feel a bit like my old self again.

(Beck, 2009, p. e6)

Interestingly, this mother "kind of liked" breastfeeding with a second baby. Some mothers have shared with me that they never liked breastfeeding but learned to tolerate it, and that was good enough. I asked why they wanted to continue. They said because it was important. It became a goal for them. As care providers, it is important that we be open to the whole range of reactions that mothers may have and support them in their decisions to breastfeed, to pump and feed their milk, or to simply formula-feed.

Breastfeeding Protects Trauma Survivors

Researchers have made some surprising discoveries about breastfeeding's effects for trauma survivors. If they can do it, breastfeeding protects their mental health and significantly lessens the risk that they will abuse their own children, something many trauma survivors worry about.

In a 15-year longitudinal study of 7,223 Australian mother–infant pairs, breastfeeding substantially lowered the risk of maternal-perpetrated child maltreatment (Strathearn et al., 2009). There were over 500 substantiated cases of maternal-perpetrated physical abuse and neglect. If mothers breastfed 4 months or longer, they were 2.6 times less likely to physically abuse their children and 3.8 times less likely to neglect them compared to mothers who did not breastfeed.

Breastfeeding also attenuates trauma, which causes a hyperactive response to stress. When stressed, trauma survivors' stress system overreacts and can cause sleep problems, depression, and anger. We found that breastfeeding, because it downregulates the stress system, helps with all these symptoms. In our sample of 6,410 new mothers, 994 women had been raped (Kendall-Tackett et al., 2013). Consistent with previous studies, rape had a pervasive negative effect. Mothers slept poorly and were more tired, anxious, angry, and depressed. When we added feeding method to our analyses (feeding method X sexual assault status), breastfeeding attenuated (lessened) the effects of sexual assault.[4] Assaulted and non-assaulted women had the same rate of exclusive breastfeeding (78% for both). In our earlier analysis, exclusively breastfeeding mothers got more sleep, took fewer minutes to get to sleep, and had more daily energy than women who mixed- or formula-fed (Kendall-Tackett et al., 2011). We found that sexual assault negatively affected sleep and well-being. However, exclusively breastfeeding attenuated the effects of sexual assault, likely because oxytocin suppressed the hyperactive stress response (see Figure 6.1). What follows are three measures: total hours of sleep, depression, and anger and irritability.

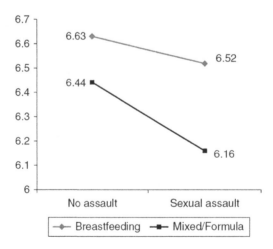

Figure 6.1 Exclusive breastfeeding's effects on total hours mothers sleep.

Source: Kendall-Tackett et al. (2013).

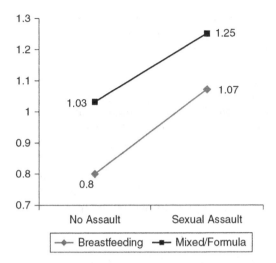

Figure 6.2 Sexually assaulted women had increased risk of depression, but exclusive breastfeeding attenuated that effect.

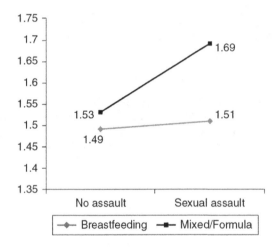

Figure 6.3 Exclusive breastfeeding lowered women's anger and irritability.

Exclusively breastfeeding mothers report more sleep (see Figure 6.2). It is somewhat less for the sexual assault survivors, but still significantly more than both non-assaulted groups.

The effects are similar with depression. Exclusively breastfeeding sexual assault survivors are still at higher risk for depression than non-assaulted women. However, they reported significantly less depression than assault survivors who are not exclusively breastfeeding (see Figure 6.3).

Sexual assault survivors reported significantly less anger and irritability if they were exclusively breastfeeding. For assault survivors who were not, their response reflects a hyperreactive stress response that is common in trauma survivors. This finding, perhaps more than all the others, shows how breastfeeding downregulates an overactive stress response. Breastfeeding's powerful effect attenuated it and made it indistinguishable from that of non-assaulted exclusively breastfeeding mothers.

Clinical Takeaways

- It is important to respect mothers' breastfeeding goals and intentions because if they stop before they planned to, they are more likely to get depressed.
- If mothers are experiencing pain or struggling with milk supply, they need referrals for skilled lactation care.
- Many women who have experienced significant trauma want to breastfeed. It is important to support their goals, perhaps coordinating with a lactation care provider. Discouraging mothers undermines their autonomy and increases their risk for depression.

Notes

1 There has been some confusion in the lactation field about the definition of "breastfeeding." The articles cited in this chapter use the term in the traditional sense: the mother making milk, and the baby suckling at the mother's breast. Other variations have not been studied, but mothers who are exclusively pumping, or mothers not breastfeeding but doing skin-to-skin contact, get some of these same effects. Uvnas-Moberg, K., Ekstrom-Bergstrom, A., Buckley, S., Massarotti, C., Pajalic, Z., Luegmair, K., Kotiowska, A., Lengier, L., Olza, I., Grylka-Baeschlin, S., Leahy-Warren, P., Hadjigeorgiu, E., Valliarmea, S., & Dencker, A. (2020). Maternal plasma levels of oxytocin during breastfeeding. *PLoS One*, 15(8), e0235806. https://doi.org/10.1371/journal.pone.0235806
2 US National Health and Nutrition Examination Survey.
3 Pregnancy Risk Assessment Monitoring System (from the Centers for Disease Control and Prevention).
4 There was no significant difference between mixed- and exclusively formula-feeding mothers on any of the variables in a previous analysis, so we combined these two groups. Kendall-Tackett, K. A., Cong, Z., & Hale, T. W. (2011). The effect of feeding method on sleep duration, maternal well-being, and postpartum depression. *Clinical Lactation*, 2(2), 22–26.

Section III

Physiological Risk Factors

7 Mother–Infant Sleep and the Effect of Feeding Method

Sleep deprivation and fatigue are major challenges for new parents. While most new mothers are tired, practitioners need to watch for signs of overwhelming fatigue: a difference I describe as "tired" vs "more tired." We should always take mothers' reports of fatigue seriously, but severe fatigue is often more relevant for mental health. Yet all too often, medical practitioners ignore this important symptom, chalking it up to "normal new motherhood fatigue," and do not ask any follow-up questions.

Fatigue can decrease women's enjoyment of motherhood and ability to care for their babies and dramatically increase their risk for depression (Corwin & Arbour, 2007). This chapter summarizes current research on sleep, fatigue, and depression but also describes research on the effect of feeding method on sleep. We cannot accurately discuss postpartum sleep without considering how babies are fed. Further, based on this research, in my opinion, practitioners should not intervene with mothers' sleep without considering feeding method. *When practitioners, or family members, urge mothers to supplement to "get more rest," or encourage her to sleep away from her baby, they directly undermine nature's protections for mothers' mental health.*

What I suggest may run completely counter to all the training practitioners receive. However, two decades' worth of research all points in the same direction. This first section describes the link between sleep disturbance, fatigue, and depression without feeding method. The second section describes how feeding method influences every aspect of mothers' sleep.

KEY FINDINGS

- Sleep problems and fatigue increase the risk of depression, and depression changes sleep architecture, which increases sleep problems and fatigue.
- Sleep problems increase inflammation.
- Trouble falling asleep can be a key symptom of depression: 20 minutes to fall asleep means low risk of depression, whereas 25 minutes or longer is associated with increased risk.
- Exclusive breastfeeding improves sleep, which protects mothers' mental health, while mixed and formula feeding do not.
- Supplementation increases mothers' risk of both depression and fatigue.
- Mothers who are not exclusively breastfeeding but are bedsharing have worse mental health outcomes than any other group.

DOI: 10.4324/9781003411246-10

Sleep Problems Increase the Risk of Depression

In a study of 245 pregnant women, sleep problems were the strongest predictor of poorer health-related quality of life (Da Costa et al., 2010). Sleep problems also predicted new-onset depression and anxiety disorders in a study of 116 women at 6 months, even after controlling for prenatal anxiety and depression (Okun et al., 2018).

A study from Israel assessed 215 mothers to see if prenatal depression predicted depression and anxiety at 18 months (Gueron-Sela et al., 2021). Mothers' short sleep duration, as measured via actigraph and sleep diary, predicted moderate to high comorbidity. Short sleep perpetuated, rather than triggered, depression, possibly because it activated the inflammatory response system.

A study of 122 women at risk for depression found that sleep problems at 6 weeks predicted higher depression scores at 7 months (Lewis et al., 2018). Problems included longer sleep latency (time to get to sleep), more daytime dysfunction, and rating their sleep quality as poor. However, sleep duration, sleep disturbance, sleep efficiency, or sleep medications did not predict depressive symptoms. The researchers felt, because their study was longitudinal, they could say the poor sleep caused depression.

Sleep disturbance, fatigue, and depression were also strongly related in a systematic review of 13 studies (Bhatti & Richards, 2015). The effect sizes ranged from moderate to large. The samples were predominantly educated, middle class, older than 30, and White. In another systematic review of 35 studies, there was a strong correlation between fatigue and depressive symptoms in the first 2 years postpartum (Wilson et al., 2019).

A longitudinal study of 711 low-income, racially diverse couples attempted to establish causal pathways between sleep and postpartum depression (Saxbe et al., 2016). This study demonstrated the bidirectional relationship between depression and sleep. They found that depressive symptoms at 1 month caused sleep problems at 6 months, which caused depression at 6 to 12 months.

Childhood abuse doubled the risk of poor sleep quality in early pregnancy in a study of 634 pregnant women from Peru (Barrios et al., 2015). Women's risk of sleep problems increased by 2.43 times if they had been both physically and sexually abused. The more abuse experiences a woman had, the worse her sleep. Prenatal depression only partially explained these findings.

Sleep Problems Increase Inflammation

Inflammation is a plausible reason for sleep problems to cause both fatigue and depression (Kiecolt-Glaser et al., 2015). Interleukin-1β (IL-1β) was elevated postpartum and had a significant, though delayed, relationship to fatigue in postpartum women (Corwin et al., 2003). Another study found a delayed effect of inflammation with a sample of 479 women. They found that sleep duration ≤5 hours per night in the first year predicted elevated IL-6 at 3 years postpartum (Taveras et al., 2011).

Groër and Morgan (2007) studied 200 women at 4 to 6 weeks postpartum and found that depressed mothers reported more fatigue and daytime sleepiness than non-depressed mothers. They had abnormally low levels of cortisol, which is a similar pattern to that seen in chronic fatigue syndrome, chronic pain syndromes, and posttraumatic stress disorder. IL-6 levels were three times higher in the depressed mothers, but this difference was not significant because of measurement variability.

Sleep Characteristics of Depressed Mothers

Depressed mothers often have specific sleep characteristics. A longitudinal study of 124 primiparous women from pregnancy to 3 months found that depressed women had more sleep disturbance, trouble falling asleep, daytime sleepiness, and early awakening than women who were not depressed (Goyal et al., 2007). Mothers with the highest depression scores had the most difficulty falling asleep. *The author noted that trouble falling asleep was the most relevant clinical screening question to assess risk of postpartum depression.*

A Taiwanese study of 163 first-time mothers found that 50% were depressed and that depressed mothers had poorer sleep than non-depressed mothers (Huang et al., 2004). Depressed mothers had overall poorer sleep quality, took more time to fall asleep (26 minutes vs 20 minutes for non-depressed mothers), had a shorter sleep duration, and reported more daytime dysfunction.

A study of 46 mothers at 6 to 26 weeks postpartum collected data via questionnaire and wrist actigraphy for seven days (Posmontier, 2008). Half of the mothers were depressed. Depressed women took longer to go to sleep (longer sleep latency), woke more often after going to sleep, and had poorer sleep efficiency.

Sleep duration also makes a difference. In a prospective study of 112 couples, sleeping less than 4 hours between midnight and 6:00 a.m., spending more than 2 hours awake during that time, and napping less than 60 minutes during the day increased the risk of depression at 3 months postpartum (Goyal et al., 2009).

Depression Changes Sleep

Unfortunately, sleep problems and depression are mutually maintaining: sleep problems can cause depression, and depression changes sleep architecture in ways that increase fatigue. In a review of polysomnographic studies of postpartum women, Ross et al. (2005) noted that sleep differed in some distinct ways for women at risk for postpartum depression or who have current postpartum depression—reduced REM latency, increased total sleep time during pregnancy, and decreased total sleep time postpartum. *REM latency* refers to when REM sleep becomes the predominant sleep pattern over the course of the night. Reduced REM latency means that REM becomes the predominant state earlier in the nightly sleep cycle, and it essentially cuts the amount of time spent in slow-wave sleep. As a result of these sleep disturbances, women are more fatigued during the day, and they also have more bodily pain.

Sleep problems can also maintain childbirth-related posttraumatic stress. A study of 95 Italian new mothers explored the link between PTSD, sleep difficulties, and parenting stress at 3 months (Di Blasio et al., 2018). Their analysis confirmed the bidirectional relationship between maternal sleep problems and trauma symptoms: sleep difficulties maintain trauma symptoms, and trauma symptoms maintain sleep problems. Sleep problems also mediated the association between trauma symptoms and parenting stress.

Sleep, Depression, and Feeding Method

Feeding method is the final variable we need to include so we can understand the complex relationship between fatigue, depression, and sleep problems. Many assume that formula-feeding mothers get more sleep, and on the surface, this seems like a safe assumption.

Looking at our data with 6,410 new mothers (Kendall-Tackett et al., 2010), exclusively breastfeeding mothers wake more often (2.5 times vs 1.3 for formula-feeding mothers). In addition, babies of exclusively breastfeeding mothers sleep the shortest amount of time at a single stretch (5.5 hours vs 7.7). These shorter sleep times and more wakenings protect infants from sudden infant death syndrome. (A prominent theory of SIDS is that babies sleep so soundly that they cannot rouse.)

Just looking at these data, we might conclude that exclusive breastfeeding wreaks havoc on mothers' mental health. But this is where things get quite interesting. *Recent research has revealed the opposite: exclusively breastfeeding mothers get **more** and better-quality sleep—particularly when babies sleep near them.* A recent meta-analysis of 7 studies ($n = 6,472$) confirmed this. They found breastfeeding mothers slept longer than non-breastfeeding mothers (Srimoragot et al., 2022).

Exclusive Breastfeeding, Fatigue, and Depression

When I first studied sleep and depression, I fully expected a dose–response effect for breastfeeding (the more breastfeeding there is, the better the protection). That is not what we found, and our findings were consistent with others. Rather than a dose–response effect, there is a threshold effect where only exclusive breastfeeding protects. As I noted earlier, mixed feeding offers substantial benefits for both mother and baby but is not sufficient to protect mothers' mental health. Supplementation, which is often recommended to depressed new mothers, *increases* mothers' risk of both depression and fatigue.

Dorheim and colleagues (2009a) prospectively studied a group of 2,830 mothers at 7 weeks postpartum and confirmed that poor sleep was a risk factor for depression. When examining the risk factors for poor sleep, "not exclusively breastfeeding" was one of them. In other words, if mothers supplement, they get less sleep and are more likely to be depressed.

A cross-sectional study of 380 mothers from Nepal found that poor sleep quality increased the risk of depression by 3.2 times and depression increased the risk of sleep problems by 2.9 times (Khadka et al., 2020). They also found that introducing complementary feeding before 6 months increased the risk of depression by 4.7 times. The rate of postpartum depression was 19%.

A study from Japan had similar results. The sample was 1,120 new mothers who completed questionnaires at 1, 2, 4, and 6 months postpartum (Maehara et al., 2017). Infant feeding methods influenced mothers' feeding routines, sleep, fatigue, and parenting stress during the first 6 months postpartum. Mothers who exclusively breastfed fed their infants more frequently but required less time per feed than mixed- or formula-feeding mothers. Compared to exclusively breastfeeding mothers, mixed-feeding mothers had more severe fatigue and took more time to feed their babies at 1 and 2 months postpartum. Exclusively formula-feeding mothers took more time to get babies back to sleep and were more stressed than mothers in the other two groups.

A study compared sleep quality for 61 exclusively breastfeeding mothers to 44 exclusively formula-feeding mothers at 4 to 14 weeks (Tobback et al., 2017). Consistent with previous studies, subjective sleep quality was better for exclusively breastfeeding mothers, and they were less tired than formula-feeding mothers. Exclusively breastfeeding mothers work more often, but the number of night wakenings is not associated with depression risk.

Breastfeeding's Effect on Risk Factors for Depression

There are two key sleep variables that predict depression: minutes to get to sleep and total hours of sleep that mothers report. Longer sleep times and falling asleep in less than 20 minutes are associated with better mental health. In our study, exclusively breastfeeding mothers fell asleep after 19.6 minutes compared to 22.4 minutes for mixed-feeding and 27.1 minutes for formula-feeding mothers (Kendall-Tackett et al., 2011). Although the times reported for mixed- and formula-feeding mothers appeared different, post-hoc analyses revealed no significant differences between the two groups. That was true for all the variables we studied.

On the second key variable—mothers' report of the number of hours they sleep—breastfeeding mothers also do well. They sleep significantly longer than their mixed- or formula-feeding counterparts (Kendall-Tackett et al., 2011). These findings run counter to the advice mothers are often given, which is to supplement so they can sleep more. Our findings, as well as those of Doan et al. and Dorheim et al., suggest that *once a mother supplements, she gets less sleep, not more* (Doan et al., 2007; Dorheim et al., 2009a; Kendall-Tackett et al., 2011). Consistent with previous studies, we found lower depressive symptoms in the exclusively breastfeeding mothers than mixed- and formula-feeding mothers (Kendall-Tackett et al., 2011). Mixed- and formula-feeding mothers were not significantly different.

Interestingly, mothers' self-report on their total sleep time is a better predictor of depression than objective sleep measures, such as an actigraph (Dorheim et al., 2009b). Similarly, an Australian study of 45 new mothers found that perceived sleep quality related more strongly to postpartum depression than objectively measured sleep time (Bei et al., 2010). A study of 115 inner-city women from New Haven, Connecticut, found the same (Caldwell & Redeker, 2009).

Longer sleep and fewer minutes to get to sleep correlated to other measures of well-being. Exclusively breastfeeding mothers were more likely to rate their health as "excellent" or "very good" compared to mixed- and formula-feeding mothers (Kendall-Tackett et al., 2011). Poor physical health limits mothers' ability to work, participate in family life, and impacts their quality of life (McCloskey, 2022). In a study from Canada using the national cross-sectional Survey on Maternal Health (n = 6,558) found that self-reports on physical health strongly correlated with mothers' mental health (Varin et al., 2020). An online survey of 306 mothers at 0 to 12 months postpartum found that mothers were more likely to report poor health if they experienced childhood adversity and current financial instability (McCloskey, 2022). Childhood adversity had a stronger effect if mothers were not also experiencing financial hardship.

Supplementation Increases Mothers' Fatigue

I have described these findings in detail because mental health practitioners often suggest supplementing with formula to help mothers "get more sleep." This strategy is counterproductive, undermines the protective effects of exclusive breastfeeding, and does not increase sleep time, as sleep researchers Doan and colleagues (2007) described.

> Using supplementation as a coping strategy for minimizing sleep loss can actually be detrimental because of its impact on prolactin hormone production and secretion. . . . Maintenance of breastfeeding as well as deep restorative sleep stages may

be greatly compromised for new mothers who cope with infant feedings by supplementing in an effort to get more sleep time.

(p. 201)

Breastfeeding, Sleep Location, and Maternal Well-Being

There is one final variable to consider regarding depression, sleep, and feeding method: Where does the baby sleep? A high percentage of mothers around the world sleep with their babies at least part of the night. In the US sample from the Survey of Mothers' Sleep and Fatigue (*n* = 4,789), we found that nearly 60% of mothers sleep with their babies at least part of the night for the entire first year (Kendall-Tackett et al., 2010). When these mothers were asked, "Where does your baby *usually* sleep?" only about 40% indicated that their babies slept with them. However, when asked, "Where does your baby *end the night*?" 60% revealed that their babies slept with them.

A recent meta-analysis of 7 studies that included 6,472 participants found more nighttime sleep in breastfeeding vs non-breastfeeding mothers (Srimoragot et al., 2022). Co-sleeping further increased the sleeping hours in breastfeeding mothers. They concluded that breastfeeding was associated with longer nighttime sleep and that co-sleeping prolonged breastfeeding.

We also examined feeding method and sleep location in our data from the Survey of Mothers' Sleep and Fatigue (*n* = 6,410) (Kendall-Tackett, Cong, et al., 2018). We combined mixed- and formula-feeding after previous analyses revealed no significant difference between the two (Kendall-Tackett et al., 2011). The findings reveal the complex relationship between breastfeeding, sleep location, and maternal well-being. As found in previous studies, bedsharing helped sustain breastfeeding (Kendall-Tackett, Cong, et al., 2018). There was a main effect of feeding method (exclusive vs not exclusive breastfeeding). For example, exclusive breastfeeding/bedsharing mothers got more total sleep and fell asleep more quickly than their non-exclusive/non-bedsharing counterparts (Kendall-Tackett, Cong, et al., 2018). Overall, the exclusively breastfeeding mothers had lower depressive symptoms regardless of sleep location, but the exclusive/bedsharing mothers had the lowest rates of all.

Some of the more surprising findings were for mothers who were non-exclusively breastfeeding but bedsharing (Kendall-Tackett, Cong, et al., 2018). For example, these mothers took longer to get to sleep and were significantly angrier and more irritable (these mothers had the highest anger scores). We need more research on this topic, but our findings suggest that non-exclusively breastfeeding mothers should avoid bedsharing.

Does Taking the Baby Away Help?

Many of my mental health colleagues suggest that mothers avoid contact with their babies at night to get more sleep. This is one of those ideas that work better in theory than in real life. Babies who are away from their mothers often do not settle well. We know that limiting contact at night is difficult to do, but does it improve mothers' mental health? We can examine studies where the babies are not with their mothers to see if it helps. Further, if an adult (rather than the baby) decides that a baby no longer requires night feeding, the baby's growth may falter, with the possibility of failure to thrive.

As expected, if mothers are depressed, their sleep tends to be disturbed *even when the baby is not there*. We see this in a study of 253 pregnant women. Depressed women had more sleep disturbances and more depression, anxiety, and anger during the second and third trimester than their non-depressed counterparts (Field et al., 2007).

PTSD also changes sleep. People with PTSD have more stage 1 sleep, less slow-wave sleep, and higher REM density than people without PTSD (Spoormaker & Montgomery, 2008). Sleep disturbances are a core feature of PTSD, and 40% to 50% of people with PTSD have sleep problems. These mothers will have disturbed sleep no matter where the baby sleeps.

A study of mothers and fathers with infants in the NICU also showed that sleeping away from babies did not help mothers' sleep. Sleep was disturbed for 93% of mothers and 60% of fathers (Lee et al., 2007). Mothers had longer sleep latency, more nighttime wakings, and more subjective fatigue than fathers. Data were collected via wrist actigraphy and sleep diary. The total minutes of sleep were significantly lower for mothers than fathers, and mothers reported more morning and daytime fatigue.

The bottom line is that removing the baby, or having someone else provide care, does not mean mothers (or fathers) sleep more.

All New Mothers Are Tired

Finally, I want to clarify one other misunderstanding I frequently hear from both mothers and practitioners: "I breastfed, and I was tired." In my experience, this belief fuels much of the misinformation that mothers receive. In our study, *all* the mothers were tired. Our exclusively breastfeeding mothers rated their energy level as a 3 on a 5-point scale. This is still postpartum, and it is difficult. A key question is, "Would you be *more* tired if you supplemented?" The answer is yes. Mothers in the other groups reported significantly less energy and more fatigue. Supplementing to "get more sleep" is an unfortunate myth.

Clinical Takeaways

- Fatigue is an important clinical symptom in new mothers. While most new mothers are tired, severe fatigue is not normal and increases the risk of depression.
- When assessing fatigue, it is important to consider mothers' sleep practices regarding bedtimes and napping, where the baby is sleeping, and how the baby is fed. Rule out possible physical conditions (such as anemia, infection, low thyroid and vitamin D, and possible autoimmune disease). Next, suggest that mothers have their babies nearby for nighttime feeds. Supplementing makes mothers more tired and telling them to not breastfeed for a 6-hour stretch is totally counterproductive as it will likely result in a breast infection and eventually destroy her milk supply.
- A more reasonable strategy for an exhausted mother is to aim for a 4-hour stretch of undisturbed sleep. Someone must be awake for this and ready to provide care so that the baby does not wake the mother. (I suggest doing this from 8:00 p.m. to 12:00 a.m. so that the support provider can still get some sleep.) Have the baby sleep near the mother for the rest of the night. It will also help if she can nap at least 60 minutes during the day (Goyal et al., 2007).

8 Estrogen, Progesterone, and Thyroid

The oldest theory of postpartum depression is that it is caused by the sudden drop in estrogen and progesterone. Following that logic, women in the past were treated with estrogen and progesterone. We know that women undergo substantial changes in hormone levels in the immediate postpartum period, but current studies do not support estrogen and progesterone as risk factors for depression. But a small percentage of women seem to be more susceptible to those hormonal shifts.

Similarly, postpartum hypothyroidism initially showed promise as a risk factor, but it became less clear with subsequent studies. However, women with conditions such as diabetes are more prone to this effect. This chapter examines research on possible effects of estrogen, progesterone, and thyroid.

KEY FINDINGS

- Estrogen and progesterone changes do not increase the risk for depression in postpartum women, but a small subgroup may be affected.
- There is little evidence to support using hormone replacement to treat postpartum mental illness. For breastfeeding mothers, it causes significant harm in that it completely halts milk production.
- Women with diabetes or family histories of hypothyroidism are at risk for postpartum thyroiditis.
- Women with depression and a history of trauma have an increased risk of postpartum thyroid disorders.

Estrogen and Progesterone

Estrogen, progesterone, and their metabolites are the most well-studied hormones in relation to postpartum depression. However, researchers noted that the drop in estrogen and progesterone in new mothers does not explain the high rate of depression in pregnancy, or depression in fathers and adoptive mothers. Further, rates of depression, or even the baby blues, vary by country. If this was strictly biological, we would expect a nearly universal response. However, that is not the case. Compared to many mothers in industrialized countries, women in cultures where postpartum mothers are well-cared for had far lower rates (Brummelte & Galea, 2016).

DOI: 10.4324/9781003411246-11

Does the Drop in Estrogen and Progesterone Cause Depression?

Bloch and colleagues (2000) induced a postpartum-depression-like syndrome in the laboratory with non-postpartum women: those with previous postpartum depression (*n* = 8) and women without a history (*n* = 8). They used gonadotropin-releasing hormone agonist leuprolide acetate and added back supraphysiologic dose of estradiol and progesterone for 8 weeks to simulate pregnancy and then withdrew the steroids. Sixty-three percent of the women in the postpartum depression group developed significant mood symptoms when the steroids were withdrawn. In contrast, none of the comparison women were affected. The authors concluded that reproductive hormones were involved in depressive symptoms *for a subgroup of women*. Women with a history of postpartum depression may be differentially sensitive to hormonal changes, increasing their risk of depression.

Another study compared estradiol levels in pregnant women with a postpartum depression history (*n* = 7) and those with no history (*n* = 12) (Schiller et al., 2013). Estradiol withdrawal did not increase negative affect in either group. Negative mood increased *before* delivery, "which suggests that estradiol did not necessarily precipitate the onset of negative mood symptoms" (p. e9). In addition, contrary to their hypothesis, low estradiol was related to higher positive affect but did not increase in the high-risk group after birth. The authors concluded that a subgroup of women may be differentially sensitive to hormonal shifts, although their sample size was too small to draw any conclusions.

A cross-sectional study of 308 women from China measured depression and anxiety during pregnancy and at 1 month postpartum (Ahlund et al., 2009). Seventy-one percent of the women were depressed, and 58% had anxiety. Mothers had the most symptoms in the first trimester of pregnancy and at 1 month postpartum. Serum estradiol sharply *increased* in the first trimester and sharply decreased postpartum. The authors hypothesized that it was *sharp changes* in estradiol that caused depression and anxiety, *not its decrease*.

Another US study compared estradiol, progesterone, and testosterone levels in 62 women with postpartum depression and 41 non-depressed women (Aswathi et al., 2015). Depressed and non-depressed women's estradiol and progesterone did not differ at 24 to 48 hours postpartum, but depressed women had significantly higher testosterone.

Premenstrual Syndrome and Depression

Researchers examined a possible link between premenstrual syndrome and postpartum depression in a sample of 478 women (Buttner et al., 2013). There was a significant relationship between moderate to severe premenstrual syndrome and postpartum depression, even after controlling for sociodemographic factors. Not breastfeeding and mothers' history of depression were also significantly related to postpartum depression. Single marital status and non-White ethnicity also increased the risk.

A study of 166 mothers from Korea also found a link between premenstrual syndrome and postpartum depression (Aronsson et al., 2015). Fourteen percent of participants were depressed. More women with a history of premenstrual syndrome were depressed (35%) than women with no premenstrual syndrome (5%). The researchers concluded that certain women may be more vulnerable to shifts in reproductive events.

Treating Postpartum Mental Health Conditions with Hormones

When practitioners believed that low estrogen and progesterone caused depression, they sometimes used hormone replacement to prevent or treat it. Traditionally, research on hormonal treatments has been plagued by methodological issues, such as lack of double-blind trials. At first glance, these findings seem compelling, but without a blinded study design, researchers could not account for the placebo effect.

For example, Ahokas and colleagues used 17β-Estradiol to treat severe postpartum depression and psychosis. Twenty-three women with postpartum major depression were recruited from a psychiatric emergency unit (Ahokas et al., 2001). They all had low serum estradiol concentrations. Within a week of treatment with estradiol, the depressive symptoms had substantially diminished, and by the end of the second week, when estradiol levels were comparable to the follicular phase, their scores on the depression measure showed clinical recovery.

The study of psychosis was similar (Ahokas et al., 2000). There were 10 women with postpartum psychosis who all had very low levels of serum estradiol. Within a week of sublingual 17β-Estradiol, symptoms were significantly improved. By the second week, when levels were almost normal, the women were almost completely free of psychiatric symptoms.

These studies are compelling, but the studies had limitations. First, the trials were not blinded, and there was no comparison group. Did estradiol reduce symptoms, or was it the Hawthorne effect, where any intervention has positive effects because people believe that it will? These studies raise some other questions, such as what are the normal levels of estradiol for postpartum women? Presumably, most postpartum women are low in estradiol, which drops as soon as the placenta is delivered. Why do only some become depressed or develop psychosis? Is there a certain level where we start to see psychiatric symptoms?

Despite the limited evidence, some still recommend treating postpartum depression with hormones. An astonishing article recommends using estradiol to treat *breastfeeding* mothers, saying mothers may prefer it because it is more "natural" (Moses-Kolko et al., 2009). Moreover, the authors recommended that future studies examine the transfer of this hormone into breast milk. This is spectacularly bad advice. Estradiol will effectively kill a mother's milk supply because estrogen blocks prolactin, the hormone necessary to make milk. If this treatment is given early postpartum, it will not matter how much estradiol transfers into breast milk *because there won't be any* (Hale, 2021). The authors recommended that clinicians not use this treatment until "lactation is established." Unfortunately, estrogen metabolites reduce milk supply for the entire duration of breastfeeding. This treatment would harm breastfeeding with little evidence supporting it as a treatment for depression.

Hypothyroidism

Thyroid is a hormone that regulates metabolism. Researchers have been interested in its link to mental health because low thyroid levels cause a wide range of depression-like symptoms, including an inability to concentrate, fatigue, and forgetfulness. Low thyroid decreases intolerance to cold, lowers body temperature and blood pressure, and causes weight gain, puffy face and eyes, constipation, and dry hair and skin. However, thyroid is another hormone that seems to increase risk of depression in only some women.

A study of 31 women examined thyroid levels in late pregnancy and early postpartum (Pedersen et al., 2007). Thyroid was measured from 32 to 37 weeks' gestation, and all the women had normal thyroid levels. Women with lower total and free thyroxine concentrations had significantly higher depression scores at all three postpartum assessment points. The researchers concluded that women with lower thyroxine levels may be at greater risk for postpartum depression.

Another study failed to find a link between postpartum depression and low thyroid (Lucas et al., 2001). This study recruited 641 women during their 36th week of pregnancy and followed them through the first year postpartum ($n = 444$ at the 12-month assessment). Eleven percent of the women developed postpartum thyroid disorder, and none were diagnosed with postpartum depression. (Only 2% were depressed.)

The rate of postpartum thyroid dysfunction is approximately 3%, and postpartum thyroiditis (including both hypo- and hyperthyroidism) is about 5% (Corwin & Arbour, 2007; Stagnaro-Green, 2012). Although screening all mothers may not be necessary, testing severely fatigued new mothers can be helpful. Risk factors for postpartum hypothyroidism include diabetes mellitus and a personal or family history of hypothyroidism. Women with type 1 diabetes are at triple the risk of postpartum thyroiditis (Stagnaro-Green, 2012). Screening tests for hypothyroidism include TSH levels, T3, and T4.

Childhood trauma also increased risk of postpartum thyroid disorders. In a study of 103 postpartum women from Spain with major depression, 63% had experienced childhood trauma, 54% general trauma, and 27% had experienced childhood sexual abuse (Plaza et al., 2010). Among women with major depression, a history of childhood sexual abuse increased the risk of thyroid dysfunction by 5 times and increased the presence of thyroid autoantibodies by 2.5 times. In addition, women who were more than 34 years old and who had previous postpartum depression were at increased risk of postpartum thyroid disorder.

Clinical Takeaway

- Postpartum changes in estrogen and progesterone are not related to postpartum depression for most women, but a small subgroup may be affected. Research does not support hormone replacement to treat postpartum depression, and it can specifically harm breastfeeding mothers.
- While postpartum hypothyroidism does not affect most mothers, women with diabetes or a family history are at risk. In addition, depressed women with trauma histories are also at risk. For these mothers and those with severe fatigue, testing for hypothyroidism is appropriate.

Section IV

Psychological Risk Factors

9 Attributional Style, Self-Efficacy, Perfectionism, and Psychiatric History

Many psychological factors either increase women's risk for depression or increase their resiliency. These factors include their attributional style their expectations about motherhood, their self-esteem, and how competent they feel as a parent. They may also have factors that make them vulnerable, such as previous psychiatric illness, low self-efficacy, and perfectionism. Each of these increases women's risk of depression and may co-occur.

KEY FINDINGS

- Low self-efficacy is a risk factor for depression and anxiety. It is also related to breastfeeding problems, but high breastfeeding self-efficacy lowered the risk for depression.
- Perfectionism increased the risk for depression in several studies, but one did not find this link.
- Previous psychiatric illnesses likely increases the risk for postpartum depression because inflammation becomes more reactive to current stressors.

Attributional Style

People have different ways of looking at the world and understanding what happens to them. They are either "optimists" or "pessimists," and this is known as their attributional style. Pessimists are more likely to become depressed after a negative event because they maintain internal, global, and stable attributions about why negative events occur. *Internal* attributions mean that they believe they caused the negative event because of something bad in them. *Stable* attributions mean that the person feels the negative situation will never change. *Global* attributions mean that the negative event affects most areas of their lives. Barbara's story shows characteristics of the pessimistic style because she translated the nurse's and her mother's admittedly negative comments to mean that there was something inherently wrong with her.

> I hadn't handled a lot of babies. The nurse was yelling at me, saying, "What's the matter, haven't you handled a baby before?" I was offended and hurt. *All I could think of was "I'm a bad mother."* . . . When [the depression] was really bad, I thought *"I'm a bad person. I should have never had a baby, never gotten married. I'm a bad mother. I'm crap."* I talked about it all the time until others were sick of hearing about it. . . . At one point, my mom said to me "I don't know what you are worried about. One baby is no work." All I could think was *"I'm a failure."*

DOI: 10.4324/9781003411246-13

A longitudinal study from Norway of 737 mothers found that three cognitive processes, rumination, self-blame, and catastrophizing, were related to higher depression scores at 6 weeks, 3 and 6 months postpartum, but depression scores overall dropped over time (Haga et al., 2012).

Cognitive behavioral therapy was specifically designed to address these pessimistic thoughts. There have been a few studies of attributional style in relation to depression in new mothers. An Australian study of 65 primiparous women found that dysfunctional attitudes were related to depression at 6 weeks. Women with high amounts of postpartum stress or whose babies had sensitive or "difficult" temperaments were at higher risk (Grazioli & Terry, 2000). Negative thinking and thoughts of death and dying at 1 month postpartum predicted depression at 4 months in another study of 465 postpartum women (Chaudron et al., 2001). Interestingly, although breastfeeding and bottle-feeding women did not differ in their rates of depression, women who *worried* about breastfeeding were significantly more likely to become depressed than those who did not.

Prenatal worry predicted postpartum depression in a US longitudinal study of 296 pregnant women (Osborne et al., 2021). When mothers were assessed at 6 months postpartum, high prenatal worry, but not prenatal depression or anxiety, predicted postpartum depressive symptoms and increased the risk for depression by 4 times. Most of the sample had been treated for previous psychiatric illness, so worry may have tipped the balance in a group that already had a significant risk factor.

Self-Efficacy, Perfectionism, and Personality Traits

Self-efficacy is an important construct within psychology because it predicts many positive outcomes. It refers to a person believing that they have the capacity to do what they need to do to reach a goal. In contrast, low self-efficacy is related to many negative health outcomes, including depression, as this mother describes.

> The truth of the matter is that I'm ashamed. Why is it so hard for me and looks so easy for other mothers? I saw other full-time mothers always doing things better. I felt I couldn't keep up. . . . I'm used to being the best at what I do. But I felt I couldn't [function as a mother]. Especially when I look at other moms. I can't seem to understand why I can't do this. . . . I was depending on other people's expectations. Maybe even my own expectations were too high. This led to feeling down, out of control. That's when the depression really started. Doubting I could do it. It got to where I was scared to death, nervous, chest tightness, crying, not wanting to eat.

A study of 1,406 new mothers from the Netherlands were assessed at 3 weeks and 12 months postpartum (van der Zee-van den Berg et al., 2021). They found that first-time mothers had lower self-efficacy compared to multiparous women. Low self-efficacy was also a risk factor for both depression and anxiety. Excessive infant crying, which decreases mothers' self-efficacy, was also a risk factor for anxiety.

A recent study of 1,204 women from Shanghai found that 15% experienced anxiety and 23% were depressed at 6 weeks postpartum (Liu et al., 2020). The authors hypothesized that education may protect mothers because it increased self-efficacy and reduced shame.

Self-efficacy has also been applied to breastfeeding. Breastfeeding self-efficacy is when a mother believes that she can breastfeed her baby and, if there are problems, that she can get help. A study from Norway examined whether breastfeeding self-efficacy lowered risk for postpartum depression (Haga et al., 2012). This longitudinal survey of 737 mothers at 6 weeks, 3 and 6 months postpartum, also included perception of social support. Women with high breastfeeding self-efficacy had low rates of depression at all three time points. Finally, women who perceived that they had a lot of support were less likely to be depressed.

A study of 144 women from Poland had similar results. Women with high breastfeeding self-efficacy had low rates of severe depression (Kossakowska, 2018). Twenty percent of the sample were depressed. Women with the most severe symptoms had low breastfeeding self-efficacy. These findings suggest that thought processes that increase the likelihood of breastfeeding success also lower the risk for depression.

Perfectionism

In a meta-synthesis of 18 qualitative studies, Beck (2002) found that beliefs about motherhood played a large role in postpartum depression. Mothers, and professionals who care for them, often harbor the belief that motherhood brings total fulfillment to women. Women may try to be "perfect" mothers and, when they cannot, feel like failures. First-time mothers were more prone to the myth of the perfect mother, whereas multiparous women's expectations focused on trying to cope with the new addition to their families.

A study of 596 postpartum women found that all types of support lowered the risk for depression and anxiety, but friend support had the strongest effect (Arnold & Kalibatseva, 2021). Perfectionism increased anxiety, but not depression. Support moderated the relationship between perfectionism and depressive symptoms and is especially important for women with perfectionistic tendencies.

In contrast, a study from Portugal of 386 pregnant women did not find a link between perfectionism and postpartum depression (Maia et al., 2012). The researchers excluded women who were depressed in pregnancy, which likely influenced their findings. They found that self-oriented perfectionism, others' high standards, and conditional acceptance did not predict depression at 3 months and concluded that perfectionism was not a risk factor for postpartum depression.

Personality Traits

A study from Leuven, Belgium, assessed 403 pregnant women during each trimester of pregnancy, and at 8 to 12 weeks, and 20 to 25 weeks postpartum (van Bussel et al., 2009). Two personality traits predicted depression in pregnancy and postpartum: neuroticism and regulator orientation. Neuroticism describes high sensitivity to stress and encompasses anxiety, fear, moodiness, worry, frustration, jealousy, and loneliness. Women high in regulator orientation fear that motherhood will change their lifestyles and identities too much, so they are more detached during pregnancy and postpartum. The facilitator orientation only weakly correlated with depression. These women often expect a lot from themselves as mothers and are vulnerable to depression when early motherhood does not match the ideal. Depression was highest during pregnancy and decreased after birth at both postpartum points, consistent with previous studies.

Psychiatric History

Women's history of previous depression, anxiety, or PTSD can increase their risk of postpartum depression. A Canadian study ($n = 622$) found that at 8 weeks, women's psychiatric history increased risk of depression by four times (Dennis & Ross, 2006a). Family history of psychiatric disorders did not. Risk factors for postpartum depression included prenatal depression and prior postpartum depression. Forty-five percent of this sample had a personal psychiatric history, and 62% had a close family member with previous psychiatric illness.

Previous psychiatric illness may increase risk for current depression because the inflammatory response reacts more to current stressors in people with prior mental illness (Maes et al., 2001). A study of 16 women with a history of depression, and 50 without depression at 1 and 3 days postpartum, measured IL-6, sIL-6R, and sIL-1R. After delivery, IL-6, sIL-6R, and sIL-1RA were elevated in all women. As hypothesized, women with a history of depression had even greater increases in serum IL-6 and sIL-1RA in the early postpartum period than women without a history of depression. The authors concluded that major depression sensitized the inflammatory response system, increasing risk of subsequent depressive episodes.

Although previous episodes of depression increased the risk for depression postpartum, it is by no means inevitable. Mothers with previous episodes are at higher risk, so they should alert their caregivers during pregnancy, arrange for follow-up postpartum, and get extra help and support after their babies are born. Depending on the severity of the episode, prophylactic use of antidepressants may be appropriate but is not necessary in every case. Recognizing risk and taking steps to counter it can often prevent a recurrence.

Depression During Pregnancy

Depression during pregnancy remains one of the strongest risk factors for depression postpartum. In a large sample from the Netherlands ($n = 5,109$), the strongest risk factors were prenatal depression (which increased risk by 3.86 times), abuse, and having a baby with a congenital abnormality (Walker et al., 2021).

A study from Australia of 5,219 postpartum women found that 15% of mothers had depression with at least one child (Chojenta et al., 2016). Depression during pregnancy and postpartum anxiety were the strongest predictors. Other risk factors included history of depression, emotional distress during labor, and breastfeeding for less than 6 months.

Twenty-two percent of 590 pregnant women from Florence, Italy were depressed, and 13% were depressed postpartum (Giardinelli et al., 2012). During pregnancy, 25% were positive for state anxiety. Lifetime psychiatric disorders, foreign nationality, and conflict with family or partner were the strongest predictors. The risk factors for postpartum depression included depression during pregnancy and use of reproductive technologies.

Two studies from Turkey found that depression or anxiety during pregnancy increase risk of depression postpartum. The first study included 479 pregnant women, 14% of whom were depressed (Kirpinar et al., 2010). Depression or anxiety in pregnancy increased risk. The second study of 553 women had similar results (Turkcapar et al., 2015). Risk factors for depression included depression in pregnancy, previous psychiatric history or postpartum depression, and physical violence during pregnancy or postpartum.

A sample of 2,888 mothers from the Upstate KIDS (New York) cohort participated in a study of maternal depression and children's developmental delays (Putnick et al.,

2022). Nine percent of the mothers had prenatal depression, and 9% had postpartum depression. Mothers with prenatal depression had more postpartum depression and breastfed fewer months.

Clinical Takeaways

- Psychological factors, such as a negative attributional style and unrealistic expectations, can all contribute to a mother's risk of depression. Cognitive behavioral therapy or similar modality will address many of these beliefs.
- Depression in pregnancy also raises some issues about how we conceptualize postpartum depression. Depression during pregnancy is often more common than postpartum depression. If that is the case, then postpartum is not necessarily a time of unique vulnerability. On the other hand, it might be useful to conceptualize postpartum depression in life span perspective—to see that both pregnancy and postpartum are vulnerable times.
- On a more hopeful note, even with significant risk factors, depression is not inevitable.

10 Violence Against Women

Millions of women around the world have experienced violence against women (VAW). It can happen during childhood or as an adult, and it increases the risk of depression, anxiety, PTSD, substance use, and a whole range of challenges. A qualitative study of 27 pregnant and postpartum women living in extreme poverty in Vancouver, Canada, who had experienced gender-based violence (Torchalla et al., 2015), most of them had addictions or were involved in the sex trade. These women had been beaten by partners, been physically and emotionally abused as children, and 77% reported past sexual abuse. What happened to these women has happened to many others.

This chapter describes three categories of violence: adverse childhood experiences, intimate partner violence, and a new category, military sexual trauma. All are strongly related to postpartum mental illness.

KEY FINDINGS

- Child maltreatment and ACEs, alone or combined with adult abuse, increase the risk for depression, anxiety, and PTSD.
- Partner violence is a strong risk factor for depression, anxiety, and PTSD and can even be a stronger predictor than depression during pregnancy.
- Partner violence can happen to any woman, but it is more common in women with social adversities (such as lower education, immigrant or asylum-seeker status, or living in poverty).
- The rates of partner violence are higher in countries where women have low resources and few rights. Many of these women are also depressed, but some show surprising resilience in the face of multiple adversities.
- Not surprisingly, women with violent partners are less likely to breastfeed. In one study, there was a direct path between violence and breastfeeding cessation and an indirect path via postpartum mental illness.
- Women veterans are at particularly high risk for depression even if they have not experienced military sexual trauma. For those who have, 77% were depressed in 1 recent study (Gross et al., 2020).
- Violence increases inflammation, which increases the risk of depression and other mental health conditions. Abuse survivors may also need anti-inflammatory treatments (such as EPA) to counter these negative effects. (See Volume 2.)
- Past and current violence can negatively affect women's parenting. But support and interventions can help. Mothers with good mental health are more competent in their parenting.

DOI: 10.4324/9781003411246-14

Adverse Childhood Experiences

Adverse childhood experiences (ACEs) include childhood physical and sexual abuse; emotional abuse; neglect (physical and emotional); witnessing parental intimate partner violence; parental mental illness, substance use, and criminal activity. The more types of ACEs people experience, the higher their ACE score, which can lead to potentially worse outcomes as adults (Anda et al., 2009).

Adverse Childhood Experiences were first identified in the Adverse Childhood Experiences Study, which included more than 17,000 patients in the Kaiser Permanente system, a health maintenance organization in San Diego, California. In this middle-class, middle-age sample, 51% of patients reported at least one ACE (Felitti et al., 1998). Participants who experienced 4 or more ACEs increased their risk for cardiovascular disease, diabetes, cancer, and overall premature mortality. This landmark study was the first that linked childhood abuse to adult organic disease. Subsequent studies have linked ACEs to many other conditions, including chronic pain syndromes (Sachs-Ericsson et al., 2009).

Interpersonal violence increased the risk of prenatal depression in women from an affluent suburb ($n = 1,509$) and from the inner city ($n = 2,128$) (Rich-Edwards et al., 2011). In the urban sample, 54% reported physical abuse, and 20% reported sexual abuse. In the suburbs, 42% reported physical abuse, and 13% reported sexual abuse, which was lower but surprisingly high given the affluence of the sample. Seventy-five percent of sexually abused women were also physically abused. Abused women were 63% more likely to be depressed during pregnancy, and the percentage increased if women were also abused as adults. This was true for both samples.

A Chinese study assessed women in late pregnancy and at 1 and 4 weeks postpartum (Li et al., 2017). Physical neglect was the strongest predictor for both prenatal and postpartum depression. The effects of ACEs were also cumulative: women who experienced more ACEs had higher depression throughout the perinatal period.

A large prospective study from France ($n = 3,310$) compared risk factors for early- ($n = 250$) and late-onset ($n = 235$) postpartum depression (Tebeka et al., 2021). Early-onset depression (up to 8 weeks) was related to childhood sexual abuse, stressful life events, personal history of depression, or co-occurring chronic disease. Late-onset depression was associated with childhood emotional abuse, stressful life events, unemployment, personal or family history of mood disorders, cannabis use, and an emergency condition during pregnancy.

A review of 43 studies found that women abused as children or adults had more lifetime depression and more depression during pregnancy and postpartum (Alvarez-Segura et al., 2014). If women experienced abuse as children and adults, their depression was even more severe, and it lasted longer. A review of 16 studies found that child maltreatment increased the risk for postpartum depression (Hutchens et al., 2017). The authors noted, however, that most of the studies were of low to moderate quality.

Memories of childhood abuse can come back suddenly, which caused this mother to experience severe depression and obsessive thoughts of harming her twin babies.

My depression started three days after birth. It came on very suddenly. . . . I had been sexually abused as a child. . . . It started with, "Oh my God. I was abused. I could abuse them." . . . I haven't done anything to hurt the kids. I first visualized my son being thrown into the fire. Then it was me throwing him in. . . . I'd have thoughts of smothering the kids with pillows. . . . Through all of this, I never neglected my children's needs, no matter how difficult. . . . No one ever questioned that I would hurt the kids. I'm the only one.

A history of childhood abuse increased the risk for intimate partner violence in a study of 1,556 pregnant women from Lima, Peru (Barrios et al., 2015). A stunning 70% of the women had been physically or sexually abused as children. Childhood physical abuse doubled the risk of depression during pregnancy. Abuse survivors had poorer overall health than non-abused women. In addition, childhood abuse increased the risk for partner violence by seven times and tripled the risk of partner violence in the past year, the topic of our next section.

Intimate Partner Violence

All around the world, women are beaten or raped by their intimate partners (Anda et al., 2007). Unfortunately, neither pregnancy nor postpartum protects women from abuse, but abuse makes them more vulnerable to depression. A sample recruited from an urban healthcare center in Philadelphia included 188 postpartum women who were assessed for mood and anxiety disorders (Cerulli et al., 2011). Current or ex-intimate partners assaulted 28% of the women, and 20% reported partner violence within the past year. Not surprisingly, women reporting IPV had more mood and anxiety disorders, including depression and panic disorder. The authors urged practitioners to realize that partner violence can cause perinatal mood disorders, and it might be happening where they least expect it.

The findings reveal a portrait of a patient that may appear in a pediatrician's office for a well-baby visit—exhausted, overwhelmed, and anxious. Without inquiry into the mother's experiences, it is easy for one to jump to a conclusion that she is only a nervous, sleep-deprived new mother. The findings suggest that the clinical picture may be more complex, however, and that careful assessment of the possible co-occurrence of IPV and mood and/or anxiety disorder is warranted.

(p. 1801)

Partner Violence and Depression

Recent data from the US PRAMS study found that 13% of mothers are depressed (Bauman et al., 2020). However, the rates of depression were much higher if there was partner violence before or during pregnancy (33%), or if mothers had depression before (29%) or during (34%) pregnancy. In New York, 884 women were followed from their first prenatal visit to 6 weeks postpartum (Silverman & Loudon, 2010). The strongest predictors of postpartum depression were physical or sexual abuse during pregnancy, a history of psychiatric disorders, and a psychiatric diagnosis at the first prenatal visit.

Partner violence was the strongest risk factor for perinatal depression in a review of 24 studies (Alvarez-Segura et al., 2014). Several studies have had similar findings. Partner violence at baseline was one of the strongest predictors of depression at 12 months in a study of 1,507 mothers from Australia (Woolhouse et al., 2015). Partner violence increased the risk of depression by 5 times in a Nigerian study of 250 mothers (Adeyemo et al., 2020). Of the 40 who reported partner violence, 65% reported verbal abuse, 28% were beaten, and 8% were raped.

A sample of 210 women from Mexico City found that 11% reported partner violence during pregnancy and 11% postpartum (Navarrete et al., 2021). Partner violence increased the risk of depression during pregnancy by 3.5 times, by 18.3 times at 6 months postpartum, and anxiety by 6 times. Women most vulnerable to partner violence had low income and education.

A study of 1,125 Canadian women found that refugees and asylum-seekers were more likely to experience violence during their pregnancies than other immigrants or women born in Canada (Gagnon & Stewart, 2014). Surprisingly, some of these women had low rates of depression, so researchers interviewed 10 mothers in-depth. All were migrants who had been beaten or raped during their pregnancies. Three factors aided in their resiliency: internal psychological resources (self-esteem, self-efficacy, hope, and optimism), social support, and systemic factors, such as day care, healthcare, legal services, language lessons, and social services. "Being in love" hindered resilience, as did repeating their story to various agencies, experiencing further violence, and trying to be strong.

A study of 426 women from Bangladesh at 6 months postpartum found that 35% were depressed and 35% were abused during pregnancy (Islam et al., 2017). Physical partner violence increased the risk of depression by 79%, sexual violence by 2.25 times, and psychological partner violence by 6.92 times. Demographic factors present a bleak picture of these mothers with high rates of severe depression: 63% of mothers with low education were depressed, 42% after childbirth complications, 40% after vaginal deliveries (but 25% after cesareans), 40% after late breastfeeding initiation (32% after early initiation), 63% with low decision-making autonomy, 55% who had a bad relationship with their mother-in-law, 70% after previous depression, and 80% after all types of IPV during pregnancy.

In Malawi, a study of 583 pregnant women found that 11% had current major depression and 21% had minor depression (Stewart et al., 2014). Risk factors for major depression were low support and partner violence. Women who were beaten by their partners were 19 times more likely to be depressed. Other factors included being unmarried; the father of the baby reacting negatively about the pregnancy; previous pregnancy, labor, or delivery complications; and lower levels of education.

A study of 500 women from Tanzania found that 19% experienced physical or sexual partner violence while pregnant, 39% reported childhood physical or sexual abuse, and 10% experienced both (Mahenge et al., 2018). Risk of depression increased 5.8 times if they were abused by a partner during pregnancy, and 2.7 times if they were abused as children. Surprisingly, given the level of violence in this sample, only 14% of the total sample were depressed.

A review of 67 studies estimated the prevalence of violence and mood disorders in the perinatal period (Howard et al., 2013). Violence during pregnancy increased postpartum depression risk by 3 times. It also increased the risk of PTSD and prenatal and postpartum anxiety. In addition, women depressed during pregnancy are 3 to 5 times more likely to be beaten by their partners.

In Iran, a study of 266 pregnant women found that 65% reported physical or psychological abuse during pregnancy (Tavoli et al., 2016). Women who reported physical abuse had more body pain and lower physical functioning and health. Women who reported psychological abuse had lower social functioning, vitality, and mental health.

Partner Violence and PTSD

Forty percent of 239 low-income pregnant American women had PTSD. They were part of a nurse home-visitation program following recent partner violence (Kastello et al., 2016). Forty-three percent reported physical, sexual, and psychological abuse within the past year. Age was the strongest predictor of PTSD; 80% of women 30 or older had PTSD, which suggests a cumulative effect of lifetime trauma. In addition, 65% of participants said that it was not partner violence that caused their PTSD but other events. Women at particular risk for IPV were unmarried, low-income, and with low education.

A study of 206 Latinas in the US found that 44% reported lifetime partner violence. Partner violence predicted PTSD symptoms at both points postpartum (Sumner et al., 2012). Another study of Latina women in the US included 92 women who had experienced partner violence and 118 women who had not (Valentine et al., 2011). The women were assessed from pregnancy to 13 months postpartum. Forty-four percent were depressed at one or more assessment points. Traditionally, prenatal depression was the strongest predictor of postpartum depression. However, partner violence was even stronger: it increased the risk for postpartum depression more than 5 times, whereas prenatal depression increased risk by 3.5 times. These same researchers found that 46% of partner-violence-exposed mothers were depressed at peak prevalence vs 25% of non-IPV exposed (Rodriguez et al., 2010).

Partner Violence and Breastfeeding

Understandably, women experiencing partner violence are significantly less likely to breastfeed, which also increases their risk for depression. A study of 217 mothers at 12 to 15 months postpartum found that 27% of the couples were violent. When couples were violent, mothers were 2.16 times less likely to breastfeed, 5.15 times more likely to use breast milk substitutes, and 2.71 times more likely to bottle-feed (Mezzavilla et al., 2021).

This is a problem worldwide. A large population study from 51 low- to middle-income countries (LMIC), which included between 95,320 and 102,318 mother–infant dyads, found that 33% had experienced IPV (28% physical violence, 8% sexual violence, and 16% emotional violence). Mothers exposed to any type of partner violence were less likely to initiate breastfeeding early and breastfeed exclusively for the first 6 months (per World Health Organization guidelines) (Caleyachetty et al., 2019). In Bangladesh, a study of 2,000 mothers found that 50% had experienced violence in the previous 12 months and that 28% had high levels of "common mental disorders" (Tran et al., 2020). Women who experienced IPV were 28% to 34% less likely to breastfeed exclusively. (It is amazing that they did any.) There was a direct path between violence and breastfeeding cessation and an indirect path via mental health disorders.

Mothers from Malawi ($n = 1,878$), Tanzania ($n = 3,184$), and Zambia ($n = 3,879$) participated in the Demographic and Health Surveys to examine the link between partner violence and breastfeeding (Walters et al., 2021). The rates of breastfeeding initiation the first hour after birth and exclusive breastfeeding were high in all three countries. However, mothers who experienced sexual partner violence were more likely to delay breastfeeding initiation and not breastfeed exclusively. Tanzanian mothers who experienced partner violence were 2 times more likely to not breastfeed at 12 months postpartum.

In a systematic review of 12 studies, 8 indicate that partner violence lowers breast-feeding intention and initiation and leads to cessation of exclusive breastfeeding in the first 6 months (Mezzavilla et al., 2018). A study of 1,200 Chinese mothers from Hong Kong found that women who experienced partner violence during pregnancy were significantly less likely to initiate breastfeeding than non-abused women, even after adjusting for demographic factors, socioeconomic status (SES), and obstetric variables (Lau & Chan, 2007).

In a recent review of 16 studies, most found that partner violence lowered breastfeeding rates, but some did not (Normann et al., 2020). They found that 4 of 7 studies found that IPV lowered breastfeeding duration, 5 of 10 found that IPV led to early termination of exclusive breastfeeding, and 2 of 6 studies found that IPV reduced breastfeeding initiation. The authors described many of these studies as fair to poor quality.

A Norwegian population study (*n* = 53,934) found that women who were physically, sexually, and emotionally abused as adults were 40% more likely to stop breastfeeding than non-abused women and had higher rates of postpartum depression (33%) than their non-abused counterparts (11%) (Sorbo et al., 2015). Women sexually abused as children were also at high risk.

Culture played a role in a study of 760 low-income, ethnically diverse women from upstate New York (Holland et al., 2017). History of violence led to breastfeeding cessation for White women, but it increased the likelihood of a breastfeeding plan and initiation for Black women.

Intervention for Mothers Experiencing Partner Violence

A recent study examined the impact of parenting confidence for 137 mothers who experienced partner violence while pregnant (Howell et al., 2021). It involved pairing first-time mothers with experienced ones to boost confidence. Sixty-seven percent were African American, 68% had experienced 4 or more childhood adversities, and 78% were depressed. Parenting confidence predicted mothers' ability to adapt during adversity. Surprisingly, depression was not related to parenting confidence.

Military Sexual Trauma

Military sexual trauma is a new addition to this book. Unfortunately, it is common for women in the military and we now know has been linked to depression, PTSD, anxiety, and adverse birth outcomes. Military sexual trauma ranges all the way from crude and offensive remarks to rape. Women's commanders or fellow soldiers are the perpetrators. Military sexual trauma's effects can be severe, even exceeding the effects of combat-related trauma.

A longitudinal study followed 620 US female veterans during pregnancy, and 452 were followed postpartum (Gross et al., 2020). In this sample, 52% reported sexual harassment and 30% reported sexual assault. Of women who were harassed, 71% were depressed compared to 41% who were not. In addition, 56% had PTSD (vs 24% of non-harassed) and 56% had an anxiety disorder. Among the women who reported sexual assault, 77% were depressed (vs 48%), 65% had PTSD (vs 30%), and 60% had anxiety disorders (vs 41%).

Another study on US veterans included 911 women who delivered a baby after entering the military (Nillni et al., 2020). Fifty-nine percent reported military sexual trauma, and 36% reported combat exposure. While in the military, 29% had a preterm birth and 45% had postpartum depression or anxiety. (Rate of preterm in the US is 10.5%.) Military sexual trauma also increased the risk of postpartum depression and anxiety. The study controlled for age at pregnancy, racial/ethnic minority status, childhood violence, and warfare exposure. Every increase on the sexual harassment scale decreased birthweight by 17 grams and increased the risk of depression by 9%.

Military sexual trauma also impacted mother–infant bonding in a study of 697 pregnant US veterans (Creech et al., 2022). Fifty-two percent reported harassment, and 30% reported abuse or rape. Military sexual trauma increased the risk of depression, and higher depression was related to poorer mother–infant bonding. The authors indicated that this study demonstrates the negative effect of adult trauma (vs child) on mother–infant bonding. The rates of depression in the military sexual trauma group were 28%.

Violence and Inflammation

Experiencing violence increases the inflammatory response, which increases the risk of depression. Kiecolt-Glaser and colleagues (2015) noted that adults who have experienced ACEs have higher IL-6 and TNF-α, lower parasympathetic activity, and greater dysfunction of the HPA axis. In addition, offspring may have experienced these changes (via epigenetics) if mothers experienced adversities while pregnant. Abuse survivors often have a hyperactive inflammatory response when faced with current stressors.

The Collaborative Perinatal Project enrolled pregnant women from 1959 to 1972. If the mother experienced adversity while pregnant or the offspring experienced childhood adversity, it increased inflammation in the offspring at the mean age of 42 (Slopen et al., 2015). Prenatal adversity increased inflammation (C-reactive protein) in the adult offspring by 3 times.

Child maltreatment was related to high C-reactive protein when offspring were 20 (Danese et al., 2007). The participants ($n = 1,037$) were part of the Dunedin Multidisciplinary Health and Development Study, a birth-cohort study of health behavior in New Zealand. Child maltreatment had an independent effect on inflammation, even after controlling for adult life stresses, early life risks, and adult health or health behavior. There was a dose–response effect: the more severe the abuse, the more severe the inflammation. At year 32, there was a similar finding (Danese et al., 2009). Adverse childhood experiences increased rates of major depression, systemic inflammation, and metabolic risk factors at age 32.

In a sample of 77 racially diverse pregnant women, childhood emotional abuse, physical abuse, and emotional neglect was associated with elevated CRP and IL-6 (Mitchell et al., 2018). Maternal obesity was one pathway by which physical abuse contributed to elevated CRP and IL-6.

The British Birth Cohort Study included 7,464 adults born in 1958 and followed ever since (Chen & Lacey, 2018). There was a graded relationship between ACEs and adult inflammation: the higher the ACEs, the more C-reactive protein and fibrinogen. Socioeconomic status and health behavior modified this effect. The researchers recommended protecting children from ACEs and supporting children through education so that they can get skilled and secure work. (ACE survivors as children often have difficulties in school.)

Violence History and Parenting Difficulties

Women with abuse histories may also have difficulties parenting, leading to problematic relationships with their children. A qualitative study of 32 Canadian mothers found that mothers worried that their abuse experiences would spill over and affect their parenting (Berman et al., 2014). The mothers went through a healing process, and it was important to grow from their pain, forget and forgive, let go of anger, and learn from the past. Without this, they could not be the mothers they wanted to be.

A sample of 131 child abuse survivors examined the effect of postpartum depression and resilience on parenting competence (Martinez-Torteya et al., 2018). Low-depression/high-resilience women had high parenting competence. However, depressed or low-resilient women had less parenting competence. Non-depressed mothers were more competent, with or without a history of abuse.

Child abuse survivors and non-abused women showed similar interactions with their babies (Sexton et al., 2017). This study of 173 mothers at 6 months found that mothers maltreated as children did not exhibit hostile or controlling interactions regardless of severity or type of maltreatment they experienced. Non-clinical maltreated women showed resilience regarding parenting quality for both low- and high-stress tasks. Many demonstrated enormous personal strength and resourcefulness. However, some mothers in this study deliberately contained their trauma so they could protect their babies. Unfortunately, these women described a range of harmful coping behaviors that included substance abuse, self-harm, and eating disorders. Even with difficulties and challenges, many were determined to create stability for them and their families. Many expressed fierce determination to not be like their mothers. But the idealized version of life with their babies was often very different from what they could provide.

Clinical Takeaways

- Violence happens in even affluent populations, but women with fewer resources are at even higher risk. I suggest that you screen all women for past and current violence as being relevant to their mental health.
- However, even if you ask directly, mothers may not report it until they trust you. So asking more than once can help. Also, having materials in your office about family violence or military sexual trauma can encourage women to talk to you about it.
- Safety planning for women in current abusive relationships may need to take precedent over treating them for postpartum mental disorders.

Section V
Birth-Related Risk Factors

11 Incidence, Symptoms, and Mothers' Experiences of Traumatic Birth

Penny Simkin's seminal study (1991, 1992) documented that women accurately remember details of their births years 15 to 20 years later. Birth experiences had lasting effects on how women felt about themselves as both women and mothers.

> The birth of a child, especially a first child, represents a landmark event in the lives of all involved. . . . No other event involves pain, emotional stress, vulnerability, possible physical injury or death, permanent role change, and includes responsibility for a dependent, helpless human being. Moreover, it generally all takes place within a single day. . . . [W]omen tend to remember their first birth experiences vividly and with deep emotion.
>
> (Simkin, 1992, p. 64)

Unfortunately, many women around the world have difficult or negative birth experiences. Some even report obstetric violence. Birth is important to women's sense of themselves. If a birth is difficult or traumatic, there will likely be sequelae. Depression and anxiety are the most common sequelae of traumatic births, but much of the literature focuses on PTSD. The next three chapters describe the range of risk factors for traumatic birth, including both objective and subjective factors. However, the strongest risk factor is women's relationships with their providers.

KEY FINDINGS

- Although a relatively small percentage of mothers meet criteria for PTSD, many have posttraumatic stress symptoms and other sequelae, including depression and anxiety, after a traumatic birth.
- Women's birth experiences can include all three types of criterion A events: death or threatened death, actual or threatened serious injury, and actual or threatened sexual violation.
- Women's subjective experiences of their births often differ substantially from how their providers see them.

Incidence and Prevalence of Traumatic Birth

The Childbirth Connections' Listening to Mothers' Survey II included a nationally representative US sample of 1,573 mothers. Nine percent met full criteria for birth-related posttraumatic stress disorder, and an additional 18% had posttraumatic symptoms (PTS)

DOI: 10.4324/9781003411246-16

(Beck et al., 2011). At first glance, 9% might not sound high, so here is a comparison group. In the weeks following 9/11, 7.5% of people in lower Manhattan met full criteria for PTSD (Galea et al., 2003). Those affected by 9/11 had lots of other symptoms, but consider this: the percentage of women meeting full criteria for PTSD after birth is now *higher* than it was following a major terrorist attack. Beck and colleagues (Beck et al., 2011) noted the following:

> In these two national surveys mothers did speak out loudly and clearly about post-traumatic stress symptoms they were suffering. The high percentage of mothers with elevated posttraumatic stress symptoms is a sobering statistic.
>
> (p. 226)

A prospective study of 933 mothers in Brisbane, Australia, found lower rates of PTSD than previous studies: 3.6% of women met full criteria for PTSD at 4 to 6 weeks, 6.3% at 12 weeks, and 5.8% at 24 weeks (Alcorn et al., 2010). However, 45% said their births were traumatic, 47% to 66% were depressed at 4 to 6 and 12 weeks, and 58% to 74% had high anxiety symptoms.

With data from a community sample in the UK ($n = 502$) and online ($n = 921$), Ayers et al. found that 3% of the community sample met full criteria for PTSD and 21% of the online sample did (Ayers et al., 2009). Sexual trauma and delivery type interacted. Women who experienced sexual trauma were more susceptible to the negative effects of assisted delivery or cesareans.

A study of 229 mothers from Flanders, Belgium, found that prevalence of PTSD symptoms ranged from 22% to 24% in the first week, and 13% to 20% at 6 weeks postpartum (de Schepper et al., 2016). Trauma symptoms dropped off quickly after 6 weeks. Women's sense of being in control during their labors protected them from birth-related PTSD.

Diagnostic Criteria for PTSD

Posttraumatic stress disorder (PTSD) is diagnosed when someone meets criteria established by the *Diagnostic and Statistical Manual-5 Text Revision* (American Psychiatric Association, 2022). Most people exposed to traumatic events do not meet criteria for PTSD. People with no symptoms are called "resilient." Some develop depression or anxiety disorders, but not PTSD. Finally, others meet full or partial criteria for PTSD. The following is a brief description of the diagnostic criteria for PTSD and a listing of possible symptoms.

Exposure to Traumatic Events

The first criterion, Criterion A, is severity of the event. DSM-5 defines a *traumatic event* as death or threatened death, actual or threatened serious injury, or actual or threatened sexual violation (American Psychiatric Association, 2013; American Psychiatric Association, 2022, #3557). Birth can include all three. People can be exposed to traumatic events by directly experiencing them, by witnessing them (and this would include the experiences of partners, labor and delivery nurses, doulas, and others in attendance), or by hearing about the traumatic experiences of a close friend or relative. Even if the event is not "medically true," at least from the doctor's perspective, it can still cause harm. For example, during labor, women might believe that they, or their babies, might die. This may not have been "true," but if they believe it, their bodies react as if. That is why women sometimes have terrible reactions to birth their providers thought were "perfect."

Lauren, a breastfeeding peer supporter in London, describes how she believed her baby had died. Her father had passed away two weeks before her baby was born. Lauren's mother was also present at the birth and thought she had witnessed the death of her first grandchild.

I was 28 when I had William. My father was very ill throughout my pregnancy and died 2 weeks before my baby was born. William was named after him and was his first grandchild. The funeral was on my due date. Fortunately, William was born two weeks late.

My labor with William was very slow. . . . I don't know how long I pushed for, but it must have been a long time as there was eventually discussion of taking me for a forceps delivery. . . . William took in a deep breath of meconium as his head turned, and my first view of him was a blue, motionless baby descending onto my chest from a great height, being vigorously ruffled on me and taken away again. I thought, "that baby is dead." That image is still what I think of when I recall his birth. . . . When he came back to me, they had put a purple hat on him. He was wide eyed, but hardly interested in breastfeeding. I thought he was brain damaged, and I still expected him to die.

. . . I don't know when I stopped expecting him to die. He was such a miserable newborn, and I remember thinking that he didn't seem to want to be alive, just as my father felt in the last weeks of his illness. He was uncomfortable to be around. At no point during my pregnancy, birth, or postnatal period was I offered any sort of psychological support.

When William was 6 months old, I . . . took bereavement counseling at my local surgery. Having someone say, "what you went through was AWFUL" gave me permission to grieve and allowed me to feel sorry for myself retrospectively. I look back on that time and can't believe we, William and I, got through it. But you do, don't you? I breastfed for almost a year.

. . . William is now a wonderfully kind and sensitive 6-year-old boy, and a great big brother to his 4-year-old sister and 1-year-old baby brother. (All back-to-back vaginal deliveries, but numbers 2 and 3 were a walk in the park!)

Amanda's experience was different. She is an American hospital–based lactation consultant whose provider sexually assaulted her during her second birth.

To my great disappointment, the birth of my first-born ended in a cesarean section. The long separation afterward took a long time to heal from. When I became pregnant with my second child, I did a lot of research and decided to plan a homebirth. Unfortunately, due to some complications with the baby's heart tones, we transferred to the hospital. When I arrived, the obstetrician on call came into the room while I was having a contraction during transition. He began yelling at me that he knew that I was only there to sue him. He told me that he was going to insert the internal monitor, or he would call the attorney and make me. I was trying to tell him "Wait, no!" but he refused. He pulled my legs open and inserted the monitor. I felt extremely violated. I began having a panic attack during labor. He didn't care what I wanted; he would do what he wanted to do because he had the power.

Symptoms of PTSD

After exposure to a traumatic event, people must have symptoms in four clusters to meet full criteria. Even if someone does not meet full criteria, they can still have PTSD symptoms.

Intrusion Symptoms

Intrusion symptoms include recurrent involuntary and intrusive memories of the event (Roberts et al., 2016). These can be flashbacks, nightmares, or just a running loop of thoughts that they cannot stop (American Psychiatric Association, 2013, 2022). For new mothers, a common statement could be something like, "every time I close my eyes, I am re-experiencing my birth" (Roberts et al., 2016). Other symptoms are intense or prolonged psychological distress and/or marked physiological reactions when something reminds them of the event. One symptom is required in this cluster.

Amanda experienced intrusion symptoms for several years after the sexual assault (described earlier) that she experienced during her birth.

> For years after the assault, I had trouble being intimate with my husband. When we tried, I would feel trapped and panicked. I couldn't go to a doctor for a long time. I hyperventilated and nearly passed out at my first postpartum check-up. Every time I thought about the birth, my hands would shake, my breathing would get ragged, and I would end up in a panic state. Yet, I was in denial. I told myself that I was overreacting. Yes, he was unkind, but I couldn't bring myself to call it anything more sinister.
>
> Finally, when referring to my birth experience, a friend called it a sexual assault. Then things began to click for me. I finally began to see a therapist, who diagnosed me with PTSD. She taught me some coping mechanisms to enable me to begin to heal. I will never be fully healed from the sexual assault, but now I call myself a survivor. I still must face the gut-wrenching panic attacks, especially near the anniversary of the assault. The worst part is my child's birthday isn't the day of complete joy that it should be. It is also the day I was sexually assaulted.

Avoidance Symptoms

Avoidance refers to avoiding people, places, and things that remind them of event. Avoidance symptoms are also common following a traumatic birth. Women may avoid everything that reminds them of their traumatic births, including doctors, medical offices, and the hospital. One symptom is required in this cluster.

Beck (2015) synthesized the results of 14 studies. Mothers described numbing symptoms, just going through the motions of caregiving, and being a shadow of their former selves. Since their infants were constant reminders of what they went through, some distanced themselves from their babies. Symptoms can also flair again during the anniversary of the trauma.

Negative Changes in Cognitions and Mood

Trauma may also bring about negative changes in mood and cognitions which have gotten worse after the traumatic event. Women must have two or more of the following symptoms.

- An inability to remember an important aspect of the traumatic event.
- Persistent or exaggerated negative expectations about themselves, others, or the world.

- A persistent distorted blame of self or others about the cause or consequences of the traumatic event. These negative beliefs can include a pervasive negative emotional state, such as fear, horror, anger, guilt, or shame.
- A markedly diminished interest and participation in significant activities.
- A feeling of detachment or estrangement from others.
- A persistent inability to experience positive emotions.

After Amanda's birth (described earlier), she said that she could not remember the doctor's name or face.

To this day, . . . I do not remember the name of this doctor or . . . his face. Every once in a while, I will look him up online to remind myself (and then can't sleep for a couple of days after), but I quickly forget again. I have been told that this is a mild form of dissociative amnesia. I am guessing that his image and name disturbs me so greatly, that my mind blocks it for protection. However, I am terrified that I will run into him unawares now that I work in that hospital system as an IBCLC. This is why I keep looking him up.

Negative changes in mood and cognition overlap considerably with depression and can directly impact how a woman feels about her baby and partner (Roberts et al., 2016). Jessica describes how she blamed herself for having a cesarean.

I feel like . . . I didn't do the things I needed to do in order to give birth—and that because it is my own fault, it's wrong for me to feel bad about it and I should just suck it up, and not feel sad that I failed, or that there is a very real possibility that I will never get to give birth in the future either, and will just end up with another C-section.

Ayers et al. (2006) found that some women who had traumatic births described how they rejected their babies immediately after birth. Many reported eventually bonding with them *in 1 to 5 years*, with avoidant or over-anxious attachment styles being the most common. This is a particularly concerning symptom and one that professionals can gently help mothers address.

Changes in Arousal and Reactivity

This symptom cluster is perhaps most characteristic of PTSD. Women must have two or more of these symptoms that worsened after their births.

- Anger, irritability, or aggressive behavior
- Reckless or destructive behavior
- Hypervigilance
- Exaggerated startle response
- Problems with concentration
- Sleep problems, specifically difficulty falling or staying asleep, or restless sleep

Jessica experienced a birth where she almost died. She felt her husband abandoned her, but also recognized that he had to go to work. She also received no help from her family. Her hyperarousal symptoms, including severe sleep deprivation, compounded the normal challenges of new motherhood. In addition, postpartum exacerbated her significant health problems.

> Even before we left the hospital, I was having severe anxiety and depression. I was beyond what the word "exhausted" implies. . . . Add to that no sleep, baby's needs, and breastfeeding, and I was barely hanging on. . . . My husband had to go back to work, or they would have fired him. They couldn't have cared less that . . . he watched his wife and baby almost die. We needed the money and he had to go. Not only did he have to work, but he also had to work extremely long, stressful hours.
>
> I was terrified to be away from him. I was already experiencing posttraumatic-stress episodes. The anxiety was worse than it had ever been in my life. I don't know what I was afraid of, but I was scared and lonely all the time. I would panic several times an hour. My body became more depleted by the day . . . the fibromyalgia I had dealt with all my life was in a full flare. I was a wreck. I was diagnosed with hypothyroidism and rheumatoid arthritis.
>
> My family was nowhere to be found. . . . They wanted to pretend that everything was fine. I was on my own all day with a newborn. I would beg my husband not to go. He had to go. . . . I realize now that it was ripping his heart out to see me so depressed and sick, and to have to leave anyway, but he left to keep a roof over our heads.
>
> I got around the house on my hands and knees, dragging my baby behind me on a blanket, because I didn't have the strength, and was in too much pain, to walk. . . . When my husband got home, I would hand him the baby without saying anything, and I would go lay down and cry. My husband was completely confused. I wanted a baby. I had a baby. Why was I mad at him? And why was I so sad? We weren't talking at all. He was hurt because I didn't understand that he was trying to take care of us financially, and I was hurt because he wasn't at home to take care of me physically.

Duration and Impairment

The final criteria are that symptoms must persist for at least 1 month and must cause significant impairment in daily life.

Clinical Takeaways

- A high percentage of women describe their births as traumatic, but providers often focus solely on whether mother and baby are still alive.
- Women can have severe impairment without meeting full criteria for PTSD. Depression and anxiety disorders are often more common.
- Acknowledging women's experiences and providing psychoeducation about trauma are both very helpful and can be the first steps toward healing.

12 Pre-Existing Conditions and Objective Risk Factors

Why are some births traumatic and others are not? I have spoken to many healthcare providers who are often quick to blame the mother. "She has unrealistic expectations of what birth is like." Or "That mother has always been so negative. Of course, she had a hard time." I have been at conferences where nurses have laughed because women had birth plans. In other words, they believed that women caused their own negative births. That belief not only disrespects their patients—it is false. *Providers' relationships with their patients are the largest determiners of birth quality*. If mothers have good relationships with their providers, they see them positively. If they do not, they are more likely to report trauma (I describe studies in the next chapter).

As you might surmise, birth is complicated. There are many new studies on birth trauma; a change that I celebrate. Mothers' prior experiences, and the interventions they experience, also determine whether the birth is positive or traumatic.

To make it easier to absorb this literature, I roughly divided it into objective and subjective factors, recognizing that that distinction is somewhat arbitrary. Mothers can subjectively experience any "objective" birth variable. I also consider mothers' pre-existing risk factors, as these also influence depression and other outcomes.

Slade (2006) proposed a model for understanding birth experiences that included predisposing (pre-pregnancy/pregnancy), precipitating (perinatal), and maintaining (postpartum) factors. These can be internal (within the individual mother), external (from the environment), and an interaction between both internal and external. Over the next 2 chapters, I roughly follow Slade's model and include some of the variables from more recent studies.

KEY FINDINGS

- Prior trauma increases the risk that mothers will experience a traumatic birth.
- Women who have cesareans or forceps-assisted births are at increased risk for depression and PTSD.
- Mothers' experiences of cesareans often vary by type: planned, unplanned/non-emergent, and emergency. Planned and emergency cesareans increase the risk of depression, but unplanned/non-emergent may not.
- Overall, women are more satisfied with their births, and have less depression, if they are attended by midwives vs obstetricians.
- Epidurals *may* increase the risk of depression, but much depends on the medication used, the length of time it was administered, and other birth interventions the mothers have experienced. But some studies found that it had an effect.
- Women who experience life-threatening complications, or are injured during their births, are at increased risk for depression and PTSD.

DOI: 10.4324/9781003411246-17

Pre-Existing Risk Factors

Pre-existing risk factors make mothers vulnerable when facing the stress of birth. A study from Montreal of 308 women found that birth PTSD was more likely if women had anxiety in pregnancy and a history of sexual trauma (Verreault et al., 2012). The women were assessed at 25 to 40 weeks' gestation, 4 to 6 weeks, and 3 and 6 months postpartum. Six percent met full criteria, and another 12% met partial criteria. PTSD was three times more common in women with a history of sexual assault.

A study of 933 women in Australia found that 46% of women in the sample described their births as traumatic, and 8% developed PTSD between 4 and 6 weeks postpartum (O'Donovan et al., 2014). The researchers found that prior trauma was the best predictor of subsequent PTSD. Trauma history was also an important factor in a study of 1,071 Israeli women with high-risk pregnancies (Lev-Wiesel et al., 2009). A mother's history of trauma, prenatal posttraumatic stress (PTS), and subjective pain during delivery increased the risk of postpartum posttraumatic stress. Prenatal depression also increased the risk of birth complications.

A prospective study of 138 women in the UK found that depression during pregnancy predicted chronic posttraumatic stress (Ford & Ayers, 2012). Mothers' sense of control, number of interventions during birth, and depression in pregnancy were risk factors for acute posttraumatic stress symptoms.

Dissociation allows someone to escape from a situation when fight or flight is not possible. It can happen to anyone during an overwhelming event when usual coping mechanisms do not work. Childhood abuse predisposed mothers to dissociation during birth in a sample of 564 primiparous women (Choi & Seng, 2016). Women dissociate during labor when they feel detached from their bodies or minds in response to a birth-related stressor.

Objective Characteristics of Birth

When I wrote the original edition of this book, objective characteristics of birth were the only ones researchers seemed interested in. Vaginal births were "good," and cesarean births were "bad." Of course, it is never that simple. Some cesarean births are great if mothers had the support they wanted, had a say in whether they had a cesarean, and it was not an emergency. Other cesareans can be quite traumatizing, if they were emergencies or against the mothers' wishes, there was no support available, and the hospital environment was hostile. Similarly, vaginal births can be empowering, positive experiences. Or mothers might describe them as a rape.

While these simple models of birth have been supplanted, there is still value in knowing the objective as well as subjective aspects of birth. These details can stay with mothers for many years. Subjective experiences of birth can color mothers' perceptions so that a birth that looks great on paper traumatized the mother. In contrast, even the most frightening birth can be okay when mothers were supported and had a say in the type of care they received.

Cesarean vs Vaginal Births

A study from Israel of 1,844 women found that 23% of mothers who had cesareans had depressive symptoms, compared to 21% for assisted vaginal, and 19% for unassisted vaginal (Weisman et al., 2010). In addition, 13% reported high levels of trait anxiety. Researchers from Iran compared 50 women who had unassisted vaginal deliveries and 50 who had cesareans (Torkan et al., 2009). Women who had vaginal deliveries had better mental health at time 1 (6–8 weeks) and physical functioning at time 2 (12–14 weeks). There were no other significant differences. Quality of life improved for both groups between time 1 and time 2.

A study of 5,332 women from the UK found that women with forceps-assisted births or unplanned cesareans had the poorest health and well-being compared to other women in the sample (Rowlands & Redshaw, 2012). Women with forceps-assisted births were more likely to report posttraumatic symptoms at 3 months and ongoing physical problems than those who had cesareans. In contrast, the women who had unassisted vaginal deliveries or planned cesareans had fewer negative sequelae following the birth. Mauri had a delivery that included both forceps and a cesarean. Her traumatic birth influenced her mental health and ability to bond with her baby.

> I went into labor naturally on Sunday. I had horrific back labor and begged for the epidural I swore I wouldn't get. The night midwife broke my water in a misunderstanding about a fetal heart rate monitor that I did not want screwed into my child's head. . . . The morning midwife called us back at 11 p.m. the Thursday before, so she wasn't especially compassionate to my situation.

After many pelvic exams that she did not want, Pitocin, and the failure of old monitors, the staff said her baby's heart rate was fluctuating. She finally got to 10 cm and pushed for an hour.

> They brought in forceps, one of my truly dreaded interventions. It felt like they were going to split my pelvis in half, and I had an effective epidural. They failed, and I spiked a fever, no doubt influenced by the number of hands inside of me over the course of this ordeal. As I was sobbing on the way the OR and begging for horizontal cuts, the OB told me not to worry, she would give me a cute bikini cut.

She wanted a horizontal cut so she had a chance to have a vaginal birth after cesarean (VBAC). By the time she woke up, she did not care about her baby at all and struggled to bond with her.

> She just didn't feel like she could be mine after all of that. At her 48-hour visit, I filled out the postpartum depression survey honestly. I felt like I was drowning. The pediatrician looked at my file, noted the C-section, and told my husband, not me, that she thought I was fine, just shaken up by the experience. I was invalidated and undermined by every person who was supposed to help me because, "the baby is healthy." I haven't been diagnosed with posttraumatic stress, but now that I'm pregnant for the second time, I'm scared to death of dealing with labor and delivery professionals.

In Taiwan, a study of 351 women found that women who had cesareans were more depressed at 3 months and had more pain at all time points up to 6 months, compared with women who had vaginal deliveries (Chang et al., 2015). At 4 to 6 weeks, 49% of the whole sample was depressed compared to 56% for the women who had cesareans. By 12 months, only 33% were depressed.

In a study of 60 women who had cesarean births, 37% described their experiences as entirely positive, but 63% reported mixed or entirely negative experiences (Karlstrom et al., 2007). Women who had emergency cesareans were twice as likely to describe their experiences as negative than women who had planned cesareans.

Three hundred and nineteen women from New Zealand said that they had experienced birth trauma. Sixty-two percent had unexpected outcomes, such as emergency cesareans (Sargent, 2015). However, the other risk factors were mostly subjective, including fearing for their own or their babies' lives (53%), poor care from the midwife or doctor (47%), poor pain management or other physical trauma (42%), and baby in the NICU (27%). Interestingly, only 4% of women identified past abuse as related to their birth trauma. Of the women who experienced poor maternity care, 45% developed a mistrust of midwives, doctors, and/or the maternity care system.

Six percent of a sample of 876 Nigerian women had PTSD at 6 weeks postpartum (Adewuya et al., 2006). Instrumental deliveries or emergency cesareans increased risk for PTSD by almost 8 times. Manual removal of the placenta increased risk by almost 5 times. The authors noted that maternity care is poor in Africa, as reflected by the high rates of maternal mortality and morbidity. Yet their rate of PTSD is comparable (or lower) than in US studies. Only 15% of mothers in this sample delivered in the hospital. Others delivered at home, primary health centers, or with traditional birth attendants. Twenty-three percent had no antenatal care.

Elective/Planned Cesareans

When researchers study cesareans, they often do not distinguish between planned vs unplanned/non-emergent vs emergency. This can make a tremendous difference in women's experiences. In our study of 6,410 new mothers, we found that mothers who had planned cesareans had the most depressive symptoms, followed by mothers who had emergency cesareans (Kendall-Tackett et al., 2015). The women who had unplanned cesareans had low depressive symptoms and were comparable to mothers with unassisted vaginal deliveries. The findings about the planned and unplanned cesareans surprised us but made sense when we considered the stress vs oxytocin systems. Mothers who had planned cesareans did not get the enormous burst of oxytocin during labor that all other mothers had (Uvnas-Moberg, 2015). Because of that, they had low oxytocin as they entered the postpartum period, which makes them vulnerable to depression. If the cesarean was an emergency, they got the burst of oxytocin, since they had a trial of labor, but also activated the stress system because either mom or baby was in danger. With the unplanned/non-emergent cesarean, mothers could be involved in the medical decision-making, have the support they wanted, and had the trial of labor to give them oxytocin. Since it was not an emergency, they did not activate the stress system so still had high oxytocin early postpartum.

A large international study randomized mothers who were expecting twins into planned vaginal vs planned cesarean conditions (Hutton et al., 2016). The study included 2,804 women from 25 different countries. Fourteen percent of both groups were depressed. Breastfeeding rates were high in both groups, and the women had similar scores on all other measures of well-being and quality of life. There was no increase in depression for mothers who had planned cesareans.

Kuo and colleagues (2014) studied trajectories of 139 women who had elective cesareans in Taiwan. The overall rate of depression and anxiety among these mothers was

27% for depression and 36% for anxiety. Depression and anxiety were highly correlated, with anxiety being more common than depression.

Delivery Preference and Expectations

A study from Norway of 1,700 mothers found higher rates of PTSD in women who preferred a cesarean but delivered vaginally (Garthus-Niegel et al., 2014). Prenatal fear of childbirth, depression, and anxiety likely contributed to this reaction. Surprisingly, women who preferred a vaginal delivery but had a cesarean did not have PTSD.

In contrast, a study of 160 women found that women who strongly preferred a vaginal birth and had a cesarean were at higher risk for depression at 8 to 10 weeks postpartum (Houston et al., 2015). The stronger the preference, the more depressive symptoms they had. By 6 months, there was no difference in depressive score based on birth preference.

Model of Care

There are two distinct models of care for maternity patients: midwifery and obstetric. The midwifery model describes birth as a normal physiological event and that women's bodies are designed to give birth. This model also uses continuous support during labor. Practitioners using a midwifery model will use medical interventions as needed but are more likely to try natural interventions first.

The obstetric model sees birth as inherently dangerous, and that women's bodies need to be modified for them to give birth. This was the rationale for interventions such as episiotomies. Practitioners are quicker to offer medical interventions, such as routine monitoring and pain medication, even when there is no immediate danger. Also, patients labor alone or with their partners, and not with practitioners. Nurses may be there but often need to tend to several patients at once.

The model of care does not always correspond to the education of the provider. For example, I have known obstetricians who practice like midwives. Conversely, I know midwives who practice like obstetricians. Nurses tend to match their approach to the people they practice with. And nurses or midwives who have witnessed or participated in traumatic births tend to be more medicalized in the way they practice (Kendall-Tackett & Beck, 2022).

A study of 281 women at 1 month postpartum in Japan compared women's perceptions of their births when attended by midwives vs obstetricians (Iido et al., 2014). Overall, women in the study rated both types of care highly, but women who had midwives rated them significantly higher and were more satisfied with their care than women who had obstetricians. Women in the obstetric group had high rates of induction, augmentation, amniotomy, and episiotomy. Women in the midwifery group had longer prenatal appointments and more individualized care. More women were breastfeeding in the midwifery group. Type of care did not influence depression scores, but women in the midwifery group had lower rates of maternity blues. There were no adverse outcomes for women in the midwives' group.

Interestingly, there are also national differences depending on which model of care is more common. In countries where the midwifery model predominates, women have lower rates of birth trauma. For example, in a prospective study of 1,224 Swedish mothers, 1.3% had PTSD, and 9% described their births as traumatic (Soderquist et al., 2009). Similarly, a study of 907 women in the Netherlands found that 1.2% had PTSD, and 9%

identified their births as traumatic (Stramrood et al., 2011). The rates in both Sweden and the Netherlands are considerably lower than they are in the US and other industrialized countries. Interestingly, providers in these countries also have lower rates of birth trauma (Kendall-Tackett & Beck, 2022).

Conversely, in countries where the status of women is poor, researchers have found higher rates of birth trauma. Providers in countries such as the US, UK, and Turkey have higher rates of birth trauma for both mothers and providers (Kendall-Tackett & Beck, 2022). It is even higher in Iran. In a study of 400 women, 218 reported traumatic births at 6 to 8 weeks postpartum, and 20% met full criteria for PTSD (Modarres et al., 2012).

Epidural Anesthesia

Epidural anesthesia is controversial. Some studies, and mothers, find it helpful and are convinced that they would never have been able to give birth without it. Other studies find that epidurals can stall birth progress, increase the risk of cesareans, and have downstream negative effects on mental health and breastfeeding. So much depends on the medication used, the amount and length of time used, and whether it provided complete pain relief. As with other interventions, epidurals have their uses, but we should not believe that something shot into the central nervous system has no effect.

This is something we investigated. In our cross-sectional study of 6,410 mothers from 59 countries, women who had epidurals had higher depressive symptoms compared to women who did not (Kendall-Tackett et al., 2015). In bivariate analyses, women who had the most common birth interventions, such as epidurals, other pain medication, or induction, had significantly higher depressive symptoms. In multivariate analysis, controlling for income, education, parity, all the birth interventions, history of sexual assault, and history of depression, only three interventions were still significantly related to depressive symptoms: postpartum hemorrhage, postpartum surgery, and epidurals.

In contrast, a study from China found that epidurals actually *lowered* levels of depression (Ding et al., 2014). This study included 214 pregnant women who were planning vaginal births. Fifteen percent of mothers in the epidural group had depressive symptoms compared with 37 mothers (35%) in the non-epidural group. Attending childbirth classes and breastfeeding also decreased depression.

Obstetric Complications

Obstetric complications and ICU admission were related to maternal PTSD at 6 to 8 weeks postpartum (Furuta et al., 2016). Women were recruited from a UK inner-city hospital over 6 months (n = 1,825). Eight percent (n = 147) experienced severe maternal morbidity, including hemorrhage, eclampsia, severe hypertension, and HELLP syndrome.[1] Fourteen percent were depressed, 6% had intrusion symptoms, and 8% had avoidance symptoms. Mothers' perceived control helps them cope during these medical emergencies. If things were explained to them, or they had a say in decisions, then they had less depression and PTSD. The authors concluded that increasing mothers' sense of control during an emergency lessened postpartum mental health complications.

Women with hypertension during pregnancy can also develop PTSD. A sample of 1,076 mothers who experienced hypertension and 372 with no history of hypertension were recruited from the Preeclampsia Foundation website (Porcel et al., 2013). Conditions related to hypertension included preeclampsia, eclampsia, and HELLP syndrome. Women who had hypertension in pregnancy were 4.46 times more likely to have PTSD.

Physical Injury

Priddis and colleagues (2013) conducted qualitative interviews with 12 women who experienced severe perineal trauma (i.e., 3rd- and 4th-degree lacerations) during their births. They identified 3 themes: (1) *the abandoned mother*, where they felt exposed, vulnerable, and disempowered (the women reported feeling disconnected from their bodies. Their broken bodies were messy, leaking, and "dirty"); (2) *the fractured fairy tale*, which describes the disconnect between their expectations of birth and life with a new baby and how it really is (this impacted their ability to mother, and their sexual identities. Despite the trauma, they were proud that they gave birth vaginally); and (3) *a completely different normal*, which is their pathway to rediscover and redefine their sense of self following their injury.

Clinical Takeaways

- While some objective factors of birth can influence women's mental health, often, their subjective experience of those interventions determines whether they will have birth trauma.
- Women can experience all types of objective birth interventions differently, depending on factors such as their consent to these procedures and their level of support.

Note

1 HELLP: hemolysis, elevated liver enzymes, low platelet count, a potentially fatal complication.

13 Subjective Experiences and Postpartum Factors

Mothers' subjective experiences of their births often predict birth trauma more accurately than objective factors. Did they feel safe and cared for? Did their providers listen? Did they believe they were in danger? In a recent study of 1,480 Danish women, negative subjective experience was the most important predictor of birth trauma (Garthus-Niegel et al., 2018).

Elizabeth described how she was treated during her first birth at a major New York City hospital. In her chart, this birth probably appears "fine," but the mother's subjective experience of it was quite different.

> I had 25 hours of labor. It was long and hard. I was in a city hospital. It was a dirty, unfriendly, and hostile environment. There was urine on the floor of the bathroom in the labor room. There were 100 babies born that day. I had to wait 8 hours to get into a hospital room post-delivery. . . . There were 10 to 15 women in the post-delivery room waiting for a hospital room, all moaning, with our beds being bumped into each other by the nursing staff. I was taking Demerol for the pain. I had a major episiotomy. I was overwhelmed by it all and in a lot of pain. I couldn't urinate. They kept catheterizing me. My fifth catheterization was really painful. I had lots of swelling and anxiety because I couldn't urinate. My wedding ring was stuck on my finger from my swelling. The night nurse said she'd had patients that had body swelling due to not urinating and their organs had "exploded." Therefore, she catheterized me again. They left the catheter in for an hour and a half. There was lots of pain. My bladder was empty, but they wouldn't believe me. I went to sleep and woke up in a panic attack. I couldn't breathe and I couldn't understand what had happened.

In Elizabeth's story, we see themes of helplessness, pain, and dissociation. This birth was still vivid when she described it to me, even though several years had elapsed since it occurred, and she had had a subsequent positive birth experience.

This section describes two important and related markers of mothers' subjective experience of birth: sense of control and relationship with her provider. I also describe postpartum factors, ending with a general discussion of human rights in childbirth.

KEY FINDINGS

- Women's sense of control during birth is an important predictor of birth trauma. If they are bullied or coerced, birth trauma is more likely. If they have a say in their care, they are less likely to have birth trauma.

DOI: 10.4324/9781003411246-18

- Women's perception of the care they received was the strongest risk factor for birth trauma. If care was inhumane or degrading or they felt out of control, they were more likely to have a traumatic birth.
- All types of post-birth pain increase the risk for postpartum depression.
- Birth trauma can make breastfeeding more difficult, but many mothers report that if they can do it, it helps heal their trauma.

Mothers' Sense of Control

Ford and Ayers (2009) found that staff support lowered mothers' anxiety, improved their mood, and increased their perceived control during labor. In a sample of 876 women from Nigeria, mothers' lack of control during labor increased their risk of PTSD by almost five times (Adewuya et al., 2006). Beck's (2015) synthesis of 14 studies found that women's "terrifying loss of control" was a key issue for women who experienced traumatic births. Women reported feeling powerless and helpless, that providers seized their bodies and they no longer belonged to them. Staff did not communicate with them, which increased their sense of vulnerability and powerlessness. They felt that they could survive only through obedience.

A prospective study of 138 women in the UK found that if mothers had support and felt in control during labor, it lowered their risk for posttraumatic stress at both 3 weeks and 3 months. These variables accounted for 16% of the variance (Ayers et al., 2016). Women with a trauma history, who had more intervention during labor, and low staff support had more posttraumatic stress. The authors concluded that one-on-one care during labor and birth maximizes positive outcomes for new mothers.

Elmir et al.'s (2010) meta-ethnography of 10 qualitative studies found that women felt out of control, powerless, vulnerable, and unable to make informed decisions about the care they received. They felt betrayed by their providers. Some agreed to procedures, such as epidurals and vacuum extractions, just to make it stop.

Women who experienced birth trauma in New Zealand (*n* = 319) reported being bullied and coerced (Sargent, 2015). One mother was "physically forced to do things against my wishes." Another said, "I was bullied into an elective C-section" (p. 7), and that her partner did not support her. Providers did not listen and mothers' concerns "fell on deaf ears." Conversations with providers were disrespectful. A midwife forced a mother to get out of bed after her birth. The mother screamed in pain and the midwife looked disgusted and left. The mother had fractured her pelvis during the birth, which took over a year to heal.

Perception of Caregiving

The actions of care providers have tremendous impact on women's experiences of birth. A systematic review of articles published in the previous 5 years found that *quality of mothers' interactions with their providers was the major risk factor for birth trauma* (Simpson & Catling, 2016). If mothers felt comfortable with their providers, there was lower risk of trauma. If their care was cold, disrespectful, or dangerous, mothers were more likely to have birth trauma.

A study of 950 Turkish mothers had similar results (Dikmen-Yildiz et al., 2017). Mothers were assessed during pregnancy, at 6 weeks and 6 months postpartum. Mothers were more at risk for birth trauma at 6 months if they were dissatisfied with their healthcare providers.

The mothers in Beck's (2015) synthesis of 14 qualitative studies described the disrespectful care they received. They felt stripped of their dignity. They and their babies were in danger. They felt degraded and disrespected, like they had been raped on the delivery table. They also felt abandoned and alone, unsupported, and offered no reassurance at a time when they were very vulnerable. They described the process of birth as cold and unfeeling, like a "piece of meat on an assembly line" (p. 4). The mothers were powerless to fix or get out of the situation they were in, and they were terrified.

Women in another meta-ethnography of 10 qualitative studies had similar comments (Elmir et al., 2010). Women described the care they received as dehumanizing, disrespectful, and uncaring. It was worse if they felt "invisible and out of control." They used phrases such as "barbaric," "intrusive," "horrific," "inhumane," and "degrading." They were distressed when large numbers of people were invited to watch their birth without their consent.

A qualitative study of 42 mothers from Sweden also found that quality of caregiving also made a difference (Tham et al., 2010). Women who reported that their midwives were nervous or not interested had more PTSD symptoms than mothers with caring midwives. Mothers in the non-care group said they were afraid and ashamed during delivery, and that there was not enough postpartum follow-up.

Postpartum Factors

Women's birth experiences can cause symptoms postpartum. Pain is particularly relevant to women's physical and mental well-being. Women's birth experiences can also make breastfeeding more difficult, which itself makes women vulnerable to depression.

Pain

After birth, women may experience pain from a variety of sources: abdominal incisions, uterine contractions, swollen or engorged breasts, cracked nipples, episiotomies or perineal lacerations, back pain and headaches from spinal or epidural anesthesia, and muscle aches and pains. This pain, although generally transitory, can be severe and frightening. When pain is treated effectively, it goes away and does not cause problems. However, when pain is ignored, undermedicated, or not treated appropriately, it can trigger a prolonged and exaggerated inflammation response, which increases the risk of depression.

A review of 19 articles on depression and pain and 11 articles on anxiety and pain found that the relationship between postpartum depression and pain was well-established (Xiong et al., 2021). The link between anxiety and pain is less well-established. A study of 72 women during the third trimester and at 3 months postpartum found that labor pain and acute pain at 6 weeks were related to depression at 3 months (Lim et al., 2020).

Mothers' history of depression or pre-pregnancy pain, or negative birth experiences, increased the risk of depression by 2 to 4 times at 8 weeks postpartum in a study of 645 Danish new mothers (Rosseland et al., 2020). In addition, pregnancy pain increased the risk of persistent pain at 8 weeks by 3.7 times.

Sixty women undergoing cesareans reported their postpartum pain levels (Karlstrom et al., 2007). Seventy-eight percent had pain that was a 4 or higher on the

Visual Analog Scale (VAS), which indicated that it was inadequately controlled. Planned vs elective cesarean made no difference. Sixty-two percent reported that pain interfered with baby care in the first 24 hours, and one-third said that it influenced breastfeeding. Negative birth experiences were more likely if mothers had emergency cesareans and higher-than-expected pain. The authors emphasized that adequate pain relief was essential to facilitate a swift recovery from surgery and emotional bonding with the baby.

Eisenach and colleagues (2008) found that severe post-birth pain, *not mode of delivery*, predicted postpartum depression. Their prospective, longitudinal study included 1,288 women who had either vaginal or cesarean deliveries. Mothers had more pain if they had cesareans or perineal lacerations. Acute pain increased to risk of postpartum depression by 3 times. Ten percent of women who had cesarean births had persistent pain at 8 weeks, which increased the risk of depression. Pain is often under-medicated because providers fear giving adequate pain medication to breastfeeding women, even though most medications are compatible with breastfeeding (Hale, 2021).

Another study examined the relationship between mothers' and her partners' fear prior to delivery and level of postoperative pain for 65 women having planned cesareans (Keogh et al., 2006). Mothers had more postoperative pain if they had negative expectations and were frightened before delivery. Partners' fear and anxiety also influenced mothers' postoperative pain. In regression analyses, mother's fear was related to partner's fear, and when mother's and partner's fears were both entered into the equation, partner's fear exacerbated mother's pain. Interestingly, the mother's fear was not related to her pain.

Breastfeeding

Not surprisingly, traumatic births can make breastfeeding more difficult and possibly undermine it completely. For example, a national survey of 5,332 mothers in England at 3 months postpartum found that women who had forceps-assisted births and unplanned cesareans had the most breastfeeding difficulties (Rowlands & Redshaw, 2012).

Some of the difficulties could be because of how breastfeeding made them feel. Mothers in Beck's study describe how breastfeeding triggered flashbacks to their traumatic births.

- The flashbacks to the birth were terrible. I wanted to forget about it and the pain, so stopping breastfeeding would get me a bit closer to my "normal" self again.
- I had flashbacks to the birth every time I would feed him. When he was put on me in the hospital, he wasn't breathing, and he was blue. I kept picturing this; and could still feel what it was like. Breastfeeding him was a similar position as to the way he was put on me (Beck, 2011, p. 306).

Physiological reasons can also make breastfeeding more difficult. Traumatic or difficult births can delay lactogenesis II, when milk becomes more abundant around days 3 to 4. A study from Guatemala found that highly stressful births increased cortisol levels, which delayed lactogenesis II by as much as several days (Grajeda & Perez-Escamilla, 2002). High cortisol blocks prolactin.

For other mothers, breastfeeding provided women an opportunity to overcome the trauma of their birth experiences and "prove" their success as mothers, as these mothers describe (Elmir et al., 2010; Beck, 2011).

- Breastfeeding was a timeout from the pain in my head. It was a "current reality"—a way to cling onto some "real life," whereas all the trauma that continued to live on in my head belonged to the past, even though I couldn't seem to keep it there (Beck, 2011, p. 306).
- Breastfeeding became my focus for overcoming the birth and proving to everyone else, and mostly myself, that there was something that I could do right. It was part of my crusade, so to speak, to prove myself as a mother (Barr & Beck, 2008; Beck & Watson, 2008, p. 233).
- My body's ability to produce milk, and so the sustenance to keep my baby alive, also helped to restore my faith in my body, which at some core level, I felt had really let me down, due to a terrible pregnancy, labor, and birth. It helped build my confidence in my body and as a mother. It helped me heal and feel connected to my baby (Barr & Beck, 2008; Beck & Watson, 2008, p. 233).

Human Rights in Childbirth

The World Health Organization, in 2014, called for reform of birthing practices, noting that many mothers worldwide received disrespectful care (World Health Organization, 2014). They noted the growing body of literature on birth trauma. WHO cited numerous problems that women have reported during their births, including physical and verbal abuse, humiliation, coercive and unconsented procedures, withholding pain medication, gross violation of privacy, and ignoring and neglecting women when they have life-threatening complications. They described these practices as a violation of women's fundamental human rights.

The WHO (2014) called for professionals to strongly focus on respectful maternity care. Quality care includes support during labor with the companion of her choice, mobility, access to food and liquids, informed choice, educating women about their rights, and what they can do if their rights have been violated. There also needs to be evaluation of these health systems to ensure that providers are accountable for the treatment they provide during childbirth.

> The surge of interest in human rights in childbirth reflects a new international consensus that respectful maternity services are critical to ensuring the health of women and babies. It also reveals the enduring universal power of human rights principles that apply to all women in all countries. A human rights approach to maternity care offers the chance to enrich relationships between women and caregivers by focusing on individual, not institutional care.
>
> (Prochaska, 2015, p. 1016)

Clinical Takeaways

- Women who have had traumatic birth experiences must acknowledge their trauma if they are ever to move past it. Trying to "just forget it" is not an effective strategy.

- Women who have not processed their birth experiences may manifest symptoms, such as depression, blunted affect, and inability to empathize with others (including their infants), helplessness, self-destructive behaviors, somatic complaints, sexual dysfunctions, marital difficulties, anger, and hostility.
- Working through trauma is difficult, but it is the only route to healing.
- The most important components of any intervention focus on helping women acknowledge and accept their experiences and helping them regain a sense of self-efficacy.

Section VI

Social Risk Factors

14 Pandemic, Disasters, and Immigration

Women do not become mothers in a vacuum. They live in families, extended families, cultures, and societies. With each type of connection, mothers can be protected from or made more vulnerable to depression. Section VI describes social variables including demographics, social support, and social policies, such as maternity leave. Recent studies, however, have expanded the definition of social factors to include world events, such as pandemics, disasters, and forced migration, the focus of this chapter.

KEY FINDINGS

- COVID-19 restrictions profoundly impacted mothers' mental health and the type of maternity care they received. Restrictions increased the risk for depression, anxiety, and PTSD, with downstream effects on breastfeeding and mother–infant bonding.
- Disasters can have a long-range effect on women's mental health. Proximity to the disaster increases the risk of symptoms.
- Immigrants are at higher risk for depression if they are new to the country, are less acculturated, or are asylum seekers.

COVID-19

The COVID-19 pandemic devastated maternal mental health. An international study, conducted in 12 languages and 64 countries, examined the effects of COVID in a sample of 6,894 pregnant and postpartum women (Basu et al., 2021). Forty-three percent were at or above the cutoff for posttraumatic stress disorder, 31% for anxiety or depression, and 53% for loneliness. Eighty-six percent were somewhat or very worried about COVID. Risk factors for anxiety and depression included accessing information five or more times a day, which doubled the risk, worries about access to medical care, and their children's well-being. The more worries mothers identified, the higher their depression, anxiety, PTSD, and loneliness scores were. Hygiene and travel behaviors did not elevate symptoms, but PTSD symptoms were associated with distancing, stockpiling, canceling doctor's appointments, and prayers. Prevention behaviors did not mitigate the negative impact of COVID-19 on mothers' mental health.

COVID-19 also impacted the quality of care that mothers received. A recent study compared 1,611 mothers who gave birth at the height of COVID-19 to 640 mothers who had given birth before (Mayopoulos et al., 2021). Mothers in the COVID-19 group had more acute stress, childbirth-related PTSD, and breastfeeding problems compared to mothers who delivered before COVID-19. They bonded with their infants less. Maternity

DOI: 10.4324/9781003411246-20

care was greatly changed during COVID-19, and these changes affected mothers' mental health and mother–infant bonding.

A similar study from Russia included 611 women who gave birth before the pandemic and 1,645 who gave birth during the pandemic (Yakupova et al., 2022). The researchers assessed postpartum depression and childbirth-related PTSD. Depression and PTSD rates were already high before the pandemic so did not increase. However, during the pandemic, obstetric violence significantly increased, particularly verbal aggression, bullying, and ignoring the needs of the birthing woman, which are indirectly related to both depression and PTSD. Seventy-three percent birthed with no support during the pandemic. The pre- and post-pandemic rates of PTSD were 17.5% vs 15%, and depression were 44% vs 46%. The number of interventions was related to their PTSD scores at both time points. COVID-19 compounded pre-existing problems with birth in Russia.

A survey of 269 women who gave birth in the US found that 6% met full criteria for PTSD and 72% had symptoms (Diamond & Colainanni, 2022). Masking during labor, changes in birthplaces, and limits on support significantly predicted PTSD. Similarly, a study of 210 pregnant and postpartum women in Poland found that stress and anxiety levels were moderate to high during COVID-19 (Stepowicz et al., 2020). Women were at higher risk if they had a history of mental health disorders, were single, or were in an informal relationship.

A study of 3,356 pregnant and postpartum women from Spain found that 47% had depression, 33% had anxiety, and 8% had PTSD symptoms (Gomez-Baya et al., 2022). Women had more symptoms if they were younger, spent more time on screens, ate fast food, used substances, talked more frequently with healthcare providers, and had higher exposure to COVID-19. In contrast, women who talked with family and friends, participated in family activities, exercised, slept well, ate healthy foods, and increased personal care were less likely to be depressed or anxious.

In Mexico City, 293 women at 4 to 12 weeks postpartum had significant symptoms due to COVID lockdowns: 39% were depressed, 46% had anxiety, and 58% reported stress (Suarez-Rico et al., 2021). Pre-lockdown rates for depression were 25% and 23% for anxiety for comparable samples. An astonishing 69% had cesareans, and 35% had adverse perinatal outcomes. Mothers who tested positive for COVID while pregnant were significantly more likely to be depressed.

COVID-19 also negatively affected maternity staff, which has an impact on care (Horsch et al., 2020). Maternity providers expressed profound misgivings about the type of care they were forced to provide.

> The unique challenges that the current COVID-19 pandemic poses places maternity staff at risk of engaging in changed practices that may be in direct contravention with evidence; professional recommendations, or, more profoundly, deeply held ethical or moral beliefs and values.
>
> (p. S142)

Natural Disasters and September 11

Natural disasters and terrorist attacks can happen at any time, in any place, and can affect pregnant and postpartum women. Experiencing disasters during pregnancy can negatively affect fetal growth (Harville et al., 2010) and mothers' mental health. In a study of 317 new mothers who survived the Sichuan earthquake, 20% had PTSD symptoms, and 10% met full criteria for PTSD. Twenty-nine percent were depressed at 8 months postpartum, which was not higher than the general population (Qu et al., 2012). Consistent with other studies, women with high exposure to the earthquake (i.e., closer to the epicenter and/or more destruction) had significantly higher rates of PTSD and depression.

Hurricane Katrina

Several studies have focused on Hurricane Katrina, a category-5 hurricane that affected the US Gulf Coast, particularly New Orleans, in 2005. One prospective study included a cohort of 288 women who gave birth in New Orleans or Baton Rouge from 2006 to 2007 (Tees et al., 2010). Depression increased the risk of PTSD by more than three times. Mothers with depression, PTSD, or high hostility were more likely to report that their infants had difficult temperaments. The authors noted that maternal mental health, not exposure to a disaster, predicted difficult infant temperament. Black women and women with lower education were more likely to have had severe experiences with the hurricane (Harville et al., 2009). Severe impact on property, injury to a family member, and feeling like their life was in danger all increased the risk of PTSD and depression.

Another study using the same sample compared PTSD and depression rates in pregnant women with high vs low hurricane exposure (Xiong et al., 2010). The researchers noted that almost the entire population of New Orleans experienced severe and chronic stressors, including relocation, discontinuity in medical care, disruption of social networks, and loss of lives, jobs, and property. Fourteen percent of women with high hurricane exposure had PTSD compared with 1% for low-exposure women. In addition, 32% of the women with high exposure were depressed compared with 12% of women with low exposure.

Unfortunately, the effects of a disaster can be long-lasting. A longitudinal study of 532 low-income mothers from New Orleans measured posttraumatic stress symptoms and psychological distress one year before Hurricane Katrina, and at 7 to 19 months and 43 to 54 months after (Paxson et al., 2010). Eighty-four percent of these mothers were African American, and 32% reported that they had a friend or relative who died because of the hurricane. Thirty percent of mothers had high enough scores to indicate "probable mental illness" at the 43- to 54-month assessment. Hurricane-related home damage was especially associated with more posttraumatic stress symptoms.

September 11th

A sample of 98 pregnant women had direct exposure to 9/11 and were assessed for salivary cortisol and PTSD (Brand et al., 2006). Mothers who had PTSD following 9/11 had lower cortisol in the morning and evening than the women who did not develop PTSD. The lower their morning cortisol levels, the higher the mothers' ratings of infant distress and negative responses to novelty at 9 months, such as loud noises, new foods, or unfamiliar people. Mothers with PTSD were more likely to say that their infants had a negative response to something new, but they did not have an overall negative temperament. The authors considered a possible epigenetic effect caused by trauma exposure during their pregnancies. Donna describes how the events of September 11 influenced her during her pregnancy and made her vulnerable to depression.

> We had a joint baby shower on September 8. September 11 was three days later. My sister was injured, and they couldn't find her for several hours. I was getting bits and pieces of information. I think my depression started then. I didn't get really bad until after delivery. . . . I've been seeing a psychologist, sometimes twice a week. We're dealing with the disappointment with my difficult pregnancy, my birth, the guilt about not being the perfect mother, September 11. My sister had severe eye lacerations, and my dad still works down there.

California birth records in the 6 months following September 11 also showed an interesting pattern. They found women with Arabic last names had twice as many low-birthweight babies as any other group (Lauderdale, 2006). These women were compared with women who gave birth one year earlier, including those with Arabic last names. The findings are consistent with the hypothesis that ethnicity-related stress during pregnancy increases the risk of preterm and low birthweight.

Immigration and Forced Migration

Women leave their countries for many reasons. Even under good circumstances, being in a new country, possibly learning a new language, culture, and set of customs, can be highly stressful. Migrating may also mean leaving support behind. Refugee women may be fleeing war or violence and may have experienced the violent death of family members, sexual violation, or possible separation from other children.

Acculturation

Acculturation refers to the cultural adaptation immigrants experience as they adapt to a new country. Acculturation can include learning the language or how to navigate essential systems, such as housing; preserving the original culture; integrating into the new society; adopting the moral attitudes of the new country; and losing feelings concerning the country of birth and people with the same cultural background (Knipscheer & Kleber, 2006). Recent immigrants, or those who have not acculturated, are at higher risk for depression.

Ahmed and colleagues interviewed 10 depressed immigrant new mothers at 12 to 18 months postpartum (Ahmed et al., 2008). These women attributed depression to social isolation, physical changes, feeling overwhelmed, and financial worries. Barriers to care included stigma, embarrassment, language, fear of being labeled unfit, and staff attitudes. Some of the factors that aided in their recovery included getting out of the house; support from friends, family, and support groups; and personal psychological adjustment.

A study from Ontario, Canada, that included 519 immigrant women found that depression was associated with living in Canada 2 years or less; perceiving their pre-pregnancy health as good, fair, or poor; pregnancy complications; perception of poor health since delivery; previous depression; and low level of support (Gannan et al., 2016). In addition, living in low-income immigrant communities was associated with depression.

Another Canadian study of 1,125 women compared the rates of postpartum depression at 1 and 16 weeks postpartum (Dennis et al., 2016). Ten percent of the entire sample was depressed. However, the rates of minor or major depression at 16 weeks were 18% for refugees, 24% for asylum-seekers, 14% for non-refugee immigrants, and 7% Canadian-born women. Of interest was their distinction between refugees and asylum-seekers, which are usually grouped together. *The results of this study suggest that asylum-seekers are at even higher risk for depression than refugees.*

Immigrant vs Native-Born

Some studies distinguished immigrant mothers from native-born. In every study, immigrant mothers were more likely to be depressed, even if they had been in their country for many years. However, mothers who were recent immigrants were more likely to be depressed than immigrants who had been there longer.

An iterative review of 8 studies found that up to 42% of immigrant, asylum-seeking, and refugee women had postpartum depression compared with 10% to 15% for native-born women (Collins et al., 2011). Another review of 18 studies (*n* = 13,749 women) found that 20% of immigrant women were depressed, which was twice the rate for native-born women (Falah-Hassani et al., 2015). Risk factors included shorter length of residence, lower level of support, poorer marital adjustment, and insufficient income.

Non-Dutch women were at higher risk for postpartum depression in a study of 5,109 pregnant women from the Netherlands (Walker et al., 2021). Other risk factors included prenatal depression, state- and pregnancy-related anxiety, unwanted pregnancy, and abuse during pregnancy. A population study of 736,988 women from Denmark classified women as native Danes or first- or second-generation immigrants (Munk-Olsen et al., 2010). First- and second-generation immigrants had higher rates of treatment for depression during pregnancy or postpartum, but the overall rate was low (504 for first-generation and 242 for second-generation). The very low rates could be because the study used chart review and only identified mothers who sought treatment, which is generally a fraction of those who are affected.

A Canadian population study (*n* = 6,237, unweighted; *n* = 74,231, weighted) compared three groups of new mothers: Indigenous, Canadian-born non-Indigenous, and immigrants (Daoud, O'Brien, et al., 2019). The rates for severe depression were 6% for non-Indigenous mothers, 11% for Indigenous, and 12% for immigrant mothers. For milder depression, the rates were 13% for non-Indigenous Canadian-born, 21% for Indigenous, and 24% for immigrants. Indigenous mothers were more likely to be younger, with less education; less likely to have a cohabitating partner; more likely to be living in poverty and experiencing abuse in the past 2 years compared to the other two groups.

A study from Israel showed a similar pattern with a stratified sample of 1,128 new mothers that included three groups: Palestinian Arab, Jewish immigrant, and non-immigrant Jewish (Daoud, Saleh-Darawshy, et al., 2019). Palestinian Arab women had the highest rates of postpartum depression (21%), followed by Jewish immigrants (9%), and non-immigrant Jewish (6%). Fifty-six percent of Palestinian Arab women reported discrimination compared to 46% of immigrant women and 19% of non-immigrants. A key finding was the interaction between multiple forms of discrimination and women's identity (Palestinian Arab, immigrant, or non-immigrant). This only affected Palestinian Arab and immigrant Jewish mothers. For Palestinian Arab mothers, those who experienced multiple forms of discrimination and high ethno-national discrimination were more likely to have postpartum depression. For Jewish immigrant mothers, ethnic discrimination increased risk by 9 times.

A study from Montreal included 5,162 pregnant women, 1,400 of whom were born outside Canada (Miszkurka et al., 2012). Fifteen percent reported partner violence, which was more common for the poorest pregnant women. Women who experienced frequent violence were much more likely to be depressed. Immigrants who were abused even once had 7 times the risk for depression. For native-born Canadian women, being abused more than once increased the risk of depression by 4.8 times.

Clinical Takeaways

- Disasters and pandemics increase the risk of depression, anxiety, and PTSD. Restrictions during COVID-19 had particularly deleterious effects. As this is a more recent event, we will not know the long-term effects of these policies for several years, but I hope that policymakers learn from these studies and will improve maternity care in the event of another pandemic.
- Immigration, particularly if forced, also has a deleterious effect on maternal mental health. Support for immigrant mothers may also include services such as language classes and help navigating housing, medical systems, and other necessities in that acculturation protects mothers' mental health.

15 Smoking, Maternal Age and Socioeconomic Status, and Maternity Leave

This chapter describes other social factors that increase risk for depression and other conditions. Maternal age, income, and education have been addressed in previous editions. Researchers know these variables well. However, I noted that smoking appeared consistently in a number of different studies, so I have included it in this chapter for the first time.

KEY FINDINGS

- Smoking has emerged as a surprisingly strong risk factor for postpartum depression. One study proposed screening for smoking as a tacit screen for depression.
- Young and low-income mothers are at highest risk for depression.

Smoking

Several recent studies have identified smoking as a risk factor for postpartum depression. Whether it *causes* depression, rather than co-occurs with it, remains to be seen. However, the results have been remarkably consistent, showing that mothers who smoke are at high risk for depression. A large sample of pregnant women from the Netherlands (n = 5,109) found that tobacco and substance use were both related to increased risk of postpartum depression (Walker et al., 2021).

PRAMS data from Illinois and Maryland (n = 4,451) indicated that 18% of mothers had postpartum anxiety. Of mothers with anxiety, 35% were also depressed (6% of the total) (Farr et al., 2014). Smoking increased the risk of anxiety by 2.3 times, and comorbid depression and anxiety by 2.9 times.

A study of women from Shanghai (n = 1,204) found that smoking during pregnancy, mother–infant separation, lower education, and breastfeeding difficulties increased the risk of depression, but not anxiety (Liu et al., 2020). In a prospective study of 236 new mothers, non-smokers were the least likely to be depressed (Mbah et al., 2013). Interestingly, there appeared to be a dose–response effect between depression and smoking: the more a mother smoked, the higher her depression score. Pregnant women exposed to secondhand smoke were also at increased risk for depression.

Postpartum depression is also related to prenatal health behaviors. A prospective cohort study recruited 664 new mothers from a US hospital at 8 weeks postpartum (Dagher & Shenassa, 2012). Smoking cigarettes at any time during pregnancy and not taking prenatal vitamins in the first trimester were related to significantly higher depression. Screening in a well-baby clinic identified 15% of mothers who were depressed

DOI: 10.4324/9781003411246-21

(Freeman et al., 2005). Depression was associated with smoking and a family history of psychiatric disorders or substance use.

Another study of US PRAMS data ($n = 134,435$) found that prenatal smoking increased the risk of postpartum depression by 41%. If women smoked only after their babies were born, depression risk increased the risk by 33%. But for women who smoked during pregnancy and postpartum, depression risk increased by 54% (Barber & Shenassa, 2021). Since universal screening for postpartum depression remains an elusive goal, the authors proposed that providers assess screen for smoking as a tacit screen for postpartum depression.

Maternal Age and Socioeconomic Status

Mothers around the world, and from every walk of life, are affected by postpartum depression, anxiety, and PTSD. But young, low-income, and frequently, ethnic-minority mothers are at particular risk. This section focuses particularly on age and income. Incidence of depression among racial/ethnic minority women is described in Chapter 2.

Maternal Age

While most research has identified young mothers at highest risk for depression, clinically, I have learned that mothers at either end of the age spectrum are vulnerable to depression. Young mothers may be more at risk for depression because they are more likely to be single or unpartnered, lower-income, with possible past or current abuse. Older mothers may have been through infertility treatments, with high-risk pregnancies and possible pregnancy losses. They may be mothers of multiples because of fertility treatments. In addition, older mothers often have more education and job status, so that they are used to being competent. New motherhood can be a shock as they feel like they do not know how to do anything.

A study of 456 postpartum Ethiopian women found that 22% were depressed (Toru et al., 2018). Young maternal age (18 to 23 years), unplanned pregnancy, child sleep problems, and poor social support increased depression risk by 3 times. Similarly, a study of 3,112 women in Pune District, India found that mothers who were less than 25 years old were twice as likely to be depressed at 6 weeks compared to their older counterparts (Doke et al., 2021).

A study of 1,507 women recruited during pregnancy from six Melbourne public hospitals found that young maternal age was one of the strongest predictors of depression in the first 12 months postpartum. Others were stressful life events, social adversity, and intimate partner violence (Woolhouse et al., 2015). In contrast, not every study found young age to be a risk factor. A study of 509 postpartum teens did not find that age, income, or other demographic included were related to depression severity (Koleva & Stuart, 2014). However, since all the mothers were young, there may not be enough range to show an effect.

Socioeconomic Status

Poverty also increases the risk of depression, and it stresses relationships, limits support and access to medical care and community resources. Poor mothers may also face food insecurity, dangerous housing or neighborhoods, and the negative psychosocial effects of being at the bottom of the social strata. The connection between poverty and depression has been found in both American samples and samples outside the US.

US Samples

MOMCare was designed to address barriers to depression care in low-income ethnic-minority women (Grote et al., 2015). Patients were screened during pregnancy and asked to participate if they were depressed. One hundred sixty-four women were randomized to either intensive maternity care (longer and more frequent maternity visits) or MOMCare, specifically designed to provide depression-care management. The MOMCare intervention improved depression severity, adherence to treatment, and remission rates. It also improved PTSD severity and generalized anxiety. Most of the women had histories of childhood trauma and significant life stresses.

In a review of 9 studies of American Indians and Alaska Natives (AI/AN) mothers, depression ranged from 14% to 30% (Heck, 2021). Mothers were more likely to be depressed if they had low income, low levels of support, adverse childhood experiences, and partner violence. Living in rural areas also limited screening and access to care.

International Studies

Low socioeconomic status (SES) is a risk factor for depression around the world. In a study of 4,879 Australian women from year 1 to year 7, 16% had persistently high symptoms of depression, which started postpartum and worsened over time (Giallo et al., 2014). Several socioeconomic status risk factors were related to high symptoms: young maternal age, a non-English-speaking family, or not completing high school. History of depression was the strongest predictor overall. Low income at baseline also predicted depression at 12 months in another study of 1,507 women from Melbourne, Australia (Woolhouse et al., 2015).

A study of 153 women from Korea found that unemployment and household income predicted prenatal depression (Park et al., 2015). Low income was also a risk factor in a Japanese study of depression at 1 month postpartum (Nishigori et al., 2020). In Nepal, a study of 195 women found that 19% were depressed at 6 months postpartum (Chalise & Bhandari, 2019). Low socioeconomic status, unintentional pregnancy, pregnancy-related health problems, and lack of husband or family support were risk factors for depression.

A study of 200 mothers from Nairobi, Kenya, found that low income was strongly associated with depression (Madeghe et al., 2016). Low income was also related to PTSD symptoms from 1 to 6 weeks postpartum in a Belgian study of 229 mothers (de Schepper et al., 2016). Other risk factors were a traumatic birth and Islamic belief (perhaps a marker for immigrant status). In addition, unemployment and low income were also risk factors for depression and PTSD in mothers who survived the Sichuan earthquake (Qu et al., 2012).

Debt is another aspect of socioeconomic status specifically related to depression. In a longitudinal study of 271 families with young children, worry about debt was the strongest predictor of depression in mothers at the initial and follow-up contacts (Reading & Reynolds, 2001). Indeed, worrying about debt predicted depression 6 months later. Other economic factors, such as overall family income, not being a homeowner, and lack of access to a car, were related to depression.

Although poverty is a risk factor and depression occurs in low-income communities, we should not assume that all low-income populations have higher rates of depression. Indeed, as I'll describe in subsequent sections, there are populations with much lower incomes that are doing things to protect new mothers. Even within a low-income population, higher relative income, social support, and high self-esteem buffer the effects of poverty.

Maternity Leave

Maternity leave is another economic factor that can influence mothers' mental health. A Canadian study of 447 mothers found that women on maternity leave, or women who were employed, had the lowest levels of depression (des Rivieres-Pigeon et al., 2001). Women home full-time were more likely to report a lack of social support and to have an unwanted or mistimed pregnancy.

A prospective study of 817 employed mothers in Minnesota assessed women at 5 and 11 weeks (Dagher et al., 2009). They found that women with demanding jobs, with little control over their schedules, had more depressive symptoms. The prevalence of postpartum depression was 5% at 11 weeks postpartum.

Clinical Takeaways

- Young and low-income mothers are at higher risk for depression. They may require more social services than other clients, such state benefits, food, and housing assistance. They may also have abusive partners, so safety planning is important.
- Peer support and parenting education improve mothers' self-efficacy and can be very helpful adjuncts to mental healthcare.
- Helping US mothers advocate for themselves to get longer maternity leaves can also be an important adjunct to mental healthcare. For mothers on maternity leave, community support can also help prevent depression.

16 Social Support

Lack of social support increases the risk of depression, especially when facing stressful life events. *Social support* relates to many factors described in the previous chapters. It increases self-esteem and self-efficacy, buffers the effects of difficult infant temperaments, alters women's attributional style, and even lowers their inflammation levels (Runsten, 2013). Any effort to prevent postpartum depression must include a strong component of social support. Lack of social support can be devastating.

> This was the first grandchild on my side. I thought everyone would come to see me. My mom did, but only after I called and asked her to come. My dad came the next day, but only for the day. . . . I was very isolated after the baby. I had no friends with babies. It was hard. . . . I thought my family would come and everyone would hold the baby. Everyone came to my house at Christmas, and they spent 6 hours in the basement playing video games. I was really hurt by that. Nobody would help me. I've really never said anything. Maybe it would have been better if I had said something.

KEY FINDINGS

- Social support prevents depression, but only if the mother perceives it as support.
- Partner support is important for mental health and breastfeeding, and non-support from partners increases the risk for depression.

What Is Support?

Social support is critical to mothers' ability to navigate postpartum, but it can be difficult to define and assess. It is more than just having people around. They need to help *that mother*. How can practitioners tell whether mothers are getting effective support?

Within the construct of social support, there are two main components: the supportive action and mothers' *perception* of the action. In other words, did it feel like support to her? Take, for example, cleaning someone's home. Generally speaking, that is a kind act. Doing it for a new mother allows her to rest and focus on her baby. However, what if the mother feels judged, where there is a silent, or even spoken, question of "Why aren't you doing this yourself?" or "I didn't have help after I had a baby; you're lucky." In this context, "help" does not feel good and can even make mothers feel judged and "lazy."

Support can take many forms. Information at just the right time. Reassurance that things are going well, or empathy when they are not. Practical help such as picking up groceries, doing the dishes, or watching the baby so the mother can take a shower. A recent

DOI: 10.4324/9781003411246-22

study on breastfeeding support is quite relevant to postpartum depression. Davidson and Ollerton (2020) reviewed 8 articles on partner support for breastfeeding. Their findings get at the fundamental structure of support: action and perception of the action. When partners offered help and encouragement, breastfeeding initiation increased, but women sometimes had negative views of "help and encouragement."

Responsiveness was the most effective kind of support and included being sensitive to women's needs, respecting her decisions, and promoting self-efficacy. If partners took mothers' needs seriously and mothers and partners acted together as a team, breastfeeding initiation, exclusivity, and duration increased. When partners offered knowledge, help, and encouragement without responsiveness, breastfeeding duration decreased. With responsiveness, women felt understood, validated, and cared for. Without responsiveness, practical support meant that they are not self-sufficient, and encouragement felt like coercion to breastfeed or meet impossible breastfeeding goals.

Inadequate Support

Inadequate support was the strongest risk factor, increasing the risk of depression and anxiety by 4.6 times in an Australian study of 1,070 women with comorbid depression and anxiety (Ramakrishna et al., 2019). Low support tripled depression risk in 596 mothers from Northern Ethiopia (Shitu et al., 2019). Other risk factors were also related to lack of support, such as not having a partner through death or divorce, or they never married, which increased risk by 3.45 times.

A study from the Canadian Maritime Provinces examined the effect of parity and infant age on maternal self-efficacy, social support, and postpartum depression and anxiety (Dol et al., 2021). Almost two-thirds had low self-efficacy, 33% had anxiety, and 20% were depressed. First-time mothers had low self-efficacy and more anxiety than mothers with more than one child. Mothers of older infants had more depressive symptoms than women of younger infants and had less social support. This suggests that support drops off after the first few weeks postpartum, increasing the risk of depression.

A prospective study found that low friend and family support, and feeling unloved by partners, increased the risk of depression at 16 weeks (Webster et al., 2000). Fifty-one percent of the depressed women had low social support compared to 32% of non-depressed women. This mother described how many people wanted to help her but inadvertently undermined her.

> Everyone was really helping with the baby but me. They were too "supportive." I know my husband wouldn't want to think that. I felt like they were taking over everything. . . . I'm a very private person. I felt like everything was exposed.

Effective Support

In contrast, social support and a positive birth lowered the risk of depression and anxiety in a sample of 1,204 from Shanghai (Liu et al., 2020). Social support and higher income protected women from the negative effects of Hurricane Katrina (Paxson et al., 2010) and partially offset the effects of partner violence in a sample of 210 from Mexico City (Navarrete et al., 2021). A Canadian study of refugees and asylum-seekers found that social support from family, friends, church, work, or school increased resilience and lowered depression risk in a group of women who had experienced many lifetime adversities (Gagnon & Stewart, 2014).

All types of support negatively correlated with depression in a sample of 1,517 women. Thirty-six percent were depressed. Sixty-eight percent were Black, and 32% were White (Pao et al., 2019). The Fragile Families and Child Well-Being Study, a study of 4,900 births from 75 US hospitals, examined why support prevents postpartum depression (Reid & Taylor, 2015). Life stress increased risk for postpartum depression, while partner, friend, and family support lowered risk for all women regardless of family type. For disadvantaged mothers, support is particularly important, as most face significant life stress. Unfortunately, stress can erode the positive effects of support. The researchers suggested that clinicians explore possible ways to mitigate stress since it is a substantial risk factor for depression, and social support alone is not enough to govern its harmful effects.

In a qualitative study of 41 Canadian new mothers, social support helped women recover from postpartum depression (Letourneau et al., 2007). Partners, friends, family, other mothers, and healthcare providers were important sources of support. Instrumental (practical) and informational support were the most helpful types. Affirmation worked best when it came from other mothers who had been depressed. Mothers preferred one-on-one support more than group or telephone support, especially in the beginning. However, as they recovered, group support helped. Joanne shared that most of her friends stayed away while she was depressed, but one friend continued to reach out.

My friends didn't know what to do. They thought I had had a nervous breakdown. Many stayed away. Even now, many are surprised that I can still function. I had one friend who was very supportive and loving continually, even though she didn't understand. She brought meals, wrote little notes. She made no demands on my recovery. My mother-in-law and husband were helpful during that time too.

Partner Support

Partner support impacts mothers' mental health in three very different groups of postpartum women. The samples were 105 middle-class White mothers, 37 middle-class mothers of premature babies, and 57 low-income African American mothers (Logsdon & Usui, 2001). Those who had partner support had higher self-esteem and lower risk of depression than women without partner support.

In contrast, when partner support is not available, mothers are more likely to be depressed or anxious. A Dutch study of 1,406 mothers found that low partner support increased the risk for anxiety, but not depression, at 3 weeks and 12 months postpartum (van der Zee-van den Berg et al., 2021). Mothers with poor marital relationships were more likely to be depressed in a study of Turkish 479 postpartum women compared to those with good relationships (Kirpinar et al., 2010). In Kenya, poor marital relationship increased the risk of depression by 2.72 times (Toru et al., 2018).

A survey of 396 Canadian new mothers found that women who were depressed at 8 weeks reported significantly less partner support than non-depressed women (Dennis & Ross, 2006b). Depressed women reported that they had more conflict with their partners, and that their partners made them angry, tried to change them, and made them work hard to avoid conflict. Shared activities, problem-focused information and assistance, and positive feedback from the partner regarding infant care decreased a mother's likeli-hood of depression at 8 weeks postpartum.

Kathy faced challenges with each of her five children. Her first husband was unin-volved and absent much of the time, which made things more difficult for her.

> My first was 9 weeks premature, in the NICU for 9 weeks. I pumped faithfully every 3 hours that whole time . . . only to bring a baby home that cried furiously at the breast. . . . I gave up. My second was only 3 and a half weeks early but was small for gestational age and cried like she was hungry and not getting enough. . . . She was up every 90 minutes screaming with reflux. My husband was absent as much as possible from our lives. My third was full term and he nursed 3 months, but finished each feed with a bottle. . . . I bonded well with him and . . . with my fourth, who never breastfed. . . . I remarried and had a full-term fifth child who had trouble moving one half of her face. . . . I pump and breastfeed, and she gets a bottle. I'm in a much better marriage. I bonded well with her.

Poor Couple Relationship Also Affects Fathers

Fathers were more likely to be depressed if there was marital strife in a study from Can-ada (de Montigny et al., 2013). The same was true for fathers in Northern Iran; marital satisfaction directly and indirectly affected fathers' depression (Barooj-Kiakalaee et al., 2022). Low marital satisfaction increased fathers' risk of postpartum depression by 40% in a meta-analysis of 17 cross-sectional studies (Wang et al., 2021).

A study of 950 couples in China found that 10% of fathers were depressed (Duan et al., 2020). The researchers hypothesized that fathers' depression was related to moth-ers' depression and marital satisfaction. Another factor was mothers' relationship with their mothers-in-law; a good relationship contributed to marital satisfaction, which low-ered the risk of depression. Conversely, a poor relationship decreased marital satisfaction and increased depression risk for both mothers and fathers. In 4.4% of couples, both the mother and father were depressed.

Depression in fathers was positively associated with depression in mothers and nega-tively associated with marital satisfaction in a study of 837 new parents from Japan (Nishimura et al., 2015).

Does Depression Affect Partner Relationships?

Up until this section, we have considered the impact of poor relationships on depression or anxiety. Low support and poorer marital relationships increased the risk for depres-sion. But could depression cause relational problems and low support?

A study compared women who were currently depressed, those with a history of depression, and those with no history of depression (Hammen & Brennan, 2002). The depressed and formerly depressed women were impaired on every measure of interper-sonal behavior, their marriages were less stable, and they had less marital satisfaction than women with no history of depression.

Similarly, depressed women reported more marital dissatisfaction than their non-depressed counterparts in a study of 80 Iranian women (Jahromi et al., 2014). Depressed women had more communication problems with their partners, and their marital dysfunction persisted even after they were no longer depressed (Roux et al., 2002).

Postpartum depression also predicted mothers' sexual dysfunction in an Australian sample of 325 women at 12 months postpartum (Khajehei et al., 2015). Depression predicted infrequent sexual activity, not initiating sex, and relationship dissatisfaction. Nineteen percent were depressed in this sample.

Does Marital Status Make a Difference?

Kiernan and Pickett (2006), using data from the UK Millennium Cohort Study (*n* = 18,533), compared four sets of parents: married or cohabitating parents, single mothers with a closely involved partner, and single mothers without an active partner. They assessed whether partnership status was related to maternal smoking during pregnancy, breastfeeding, and postpartum depression.

Smoking during pregnancy, breastfeeding, and maternal depression were more common in single mothers. Cohabitating mothers had worse health outcomes than married mothers. Among unmarried mothers, smoking was more common when women did not have a regular partner. For breastfeeding, parents with stronger relationships were more likely to initiate breastfeeding. Mothers' depression negatively affected bonding. Compared to other unmarried mothers, cohabitating mothers had the worse outcomes.

Social Capital

Support can also be studied by examining *social capital*, which refers to resources that are embedded in social networks. It includes neighborhood and social network support, partner support, and internal resources. With high social capital, women give and receive support to people whom they trust.

A study of 383 pregnant Greek women found that mothers with low social capital were more depressed postpartum compared to women with high social capital (Kritsotakis et al., 2013). Community activities can increase social capital, but for women in this study, community activities provided little support, felt burdensome, and did not lower depressive symptoms. Personal relationships provided better support than participating in activities.

Social capital protected mothers from adverse birth outcomes according to data from the 2007 Los Angeles Mommy and Baby study (*n* = 3,353) (Wakeel et al., 2013). Women who had more stress than social capital during pregnancy had higher risk of preterm birth, pregnancy complications, and lower gestational age. Conversely, women with higher social capital relative to stress were less likely to have adverse birth outcomes.

What Support Could Look Like

This final section on support is more aspirational and poses an interesting question. Namely, why do rich Western industrialized countries have higher rates of depression compared to many countries that have far fewer resources? Stern and Kruckman (1983) considered this question in their classic paper and found that some cultures were much better than others at protecting new mothers' mental health. Although these cultures differed dramatically from one another, Stern and Kruckman noted that there were some common elements, which they referred to as social structures.

Social Structures That Protect New Mothers

Many cultures have special postnatal customs, including special diet, isolation, rest, and assistance for the mothers (Eberhard-Gran et al., 2010). Unfortunately, customs that included rest and assistance for the mother have decreased since the 1950s, with some modern mothers finding these rituals old-fashioned. Since these cultural practices prevent depression, it would still help to know about them so they can be adapted for modern mothers.

We must remember that just having rituals does not automatically prevent depression. Some rituals can harm maternal mental health. To make a difference, rituals must make mothers feel cared for. If they do not, the ritual may not prevent depression. For example, the Chinese tradition of not allowing new mothers to bathe or wash their hair for a month is one that mothers find onerous, and they are happier if they can bathe. Seclusion can also make new mothers feel trapped if they do not like the people they are secluded with (Klainin & Arthur, 2009). The characteristics that Stern and Kruckman (1983) described as protecting the mental health of new mothers are as follows.

A Distinct Postpartum Period

In cultures that protect new mothers, postpartum is recognized as distinct from normal life. It is a time when mothers recuperate, their activities are limited, and they are taken care of by female relatives. "Lying-in" was also common practice in colonial America. This is like the 40-day period in Latin America, *la cuarantena* ("the quarantine"), and "doing the month" in China (Eberhard-Gran et al., 2010).

Measures That Reflect the New Mother's Vulnerability

New mothers are recognized as especially vulnerable, and many cultural rituals are associated with mothers' vulnerability. There are foods mothers must either eat or avoid. For example, in China, mothers must have a special hot postpartum tea and avoid cold foods and drinks. Postpartum porridge was common in the Middle Ages as something that guests would bring that would protect mother and child (Eberhard-Gran et al., 2010). Wrapping of mothers' head or abdomen, limitations on the amount of company they receive—all these rituals protect the mother and set aside the postpartum period as distinct from normal life.

Social Seclusion and Mandated Rest

Social seclusion is another way to protect new mothers. During this time, mothers are supposed to rest and restrict normal activities. In the Punjab, women only see female relatives and the midwife for 5 days. After the 5 days, there is a "stepping out" ceremony for the mother and baby. In other cultures, seclusion can be up to 3 months. Seclusion and rest allow mothers to recover. In Nigeria, women and infants are isolated in a "fattening room," where the mother's duty, for 2 or 3 months postpartum, is to gain weight, sleep, and care for her infant (Eberhard-Gran et al., 2010).

Functional Assistance

To ensure that women get the rest they need, someone needs to handle their normal workload. Functional assistance involves care of older children, household help, and personal attendance during labor. Women may return to their families' homes to ensure that this type of assistance is available. In Germany, *Wochenbett* (weeks in bed) means that women should not only rest but literally stay in bed during the postpartum period (Eberhard-Gran et al., 2010). Postpartum doula Salle Webber (2012) describes the care that mothers need in her book *The Gentle Art of Newborn Family Care.*

> In traditional and tribal cultures, mother and child are cared for, sheltered, and protected for up to 40 days after birth. Women of the community attend to their personal needs, and care for the home and family. Generally, the mother and infant don't leave home during that time. It is understood that this period is delicate, baby's life is tenuous, and the mother needs to rebuild her strength to feed and care for her child in the years ahead.
>
> To the tribe, each life is valuable, and they worked together to provide the best possible outcome, knowing that life can slip away quickly. With our modern medical facilities, we often fail to recall what a tremendous miracle it is to undergo a pregnancy and childbirth, and to raise a child. We expect successful outcomes, yet the possibilities of complications are vast, as our foremothers knew all too well. It is prudent to treat the postpartum weeks in a tender and careful way, as an investment in the long-term health and well-being of mother and child.
>
> (pp. 25–26)

Social Recognition of Her New Role and Status

In cultures with low incidence of the blues or depression, people pay attention to the mother and recognize her new status. For example, Punjabi culture has a ritual stepping-out ceremony, ritual bathing and hair-washing performed by the midwife, and a ceremonial meal prepared by a Brahmin. Mothers receive gifts for their babies—and themselves. Similarly, ritual bathing, hair-washing, massage, abdominal binding, and other types of personal care are also prominent in the postpartum rituals of rural Guatemala, Mayan women in the Yucatan, and Latina women both in the United States and Mexico. Here is one of my favorite descriptions of a recognition ritual performed by the Chagga people of Uganda:

> Three months after the birth of her child, the Chagga woman's head is shaved and crowned with a bead tiara, she is robed in an ancient skin garment worked with beads, a staff such as the elders carry is put in her hand, and she emerges from her hut for her first public appearance with her baby. Proceeding slowly towards the market, they are greeted with songs such as are sung to warriors returning from battle. She and her baby have survived the weeks of danger. The child is no longer vulnerable, but a baby who has learned what love means, has smiled its first smiles, and is now ready to learn about the bright, loud world outside.
>
> (Dunham, 1992, p. 148)

What 21st-Century Mothers Face

Since the 1950s, postpartum rituals have gradually died out in many industrialized countries. Hospitals once provided some of this support, but hospital stays shortened, even for cesareans, and mothers stepped immediately back into their lives. Further, once a woman had her baby, all the attention shifted to the baby (Eberhard-Gran et al., 2010). Many of the mothers interviewed for this book felt a profound sense of loss and abandonment by their medical caregivers and their families. In general, there was little acknowledgment of what these women had been through, both physically and emotionally, by giving birth. Following are what some of these mothers said.

- I really wanted someone to make me feel special. All the attention was on the baby.
- I feel a sense of anti-climax. I was used to being the center of attention. Then I had to go back to being a normal healthy person. I'm not begging for attention, but now everyone only pays attention to the baby. It would be nice to have some attention afterwards. While you're pregnant, you're feeling fat and slobby, and don't want it. After the baby, you want it.
- I felt like I didn't matter. I felt like they weren't interested in me after I had my baby. . . . My husband said "of course they are not interested. You've had your baby." The 6-week visit seemed like an eternity away. I wrote [my midwife] a note to thank her. She didn't even mention it when I saw her at 6 weeks. . . . When I felt great, they treated me nicely. Now when I feel so awful with this baby, no one seems to be available to me.
- My doctor thought her job was done after my daughter was born. It's ridiculous to think the job is done just because you've delivered the baby. I called her a couple of times after, and she told me to see a social worker. I eventually left my OB. There were many reasons, but mainly because she left me high and dry after delivery.
- After the birth, I had several people tell me that the most important thing was that I had a healthy baby. Yes, that is important. But what about me? No one pays attention to the fact that you've had major surgery. They would have paid more attention if you had had your appendix out.

Clinical Takeaways

- Social support plays a key role in preventing postpartum depression and can buffer life stress. Beyond a woman's immediate circle of family and friends, an entire culture can determine whether mothers are supported or vulnerable to depression.
- Helping mothers access support, including partner support, can be a critical part of her recovery.

Section VII
Infant Characteristics

17 Infant Crying, Temperament, and Sleep

Infant crying and sleep can profoundly affect maternal mental health. For many years, the relationship between infant crying and maternal depression seemed straightforward: the more babies cried, the higher the mothers' risk for depression. For example, mothers of babies who excessively cry or refuse to feed were more likely to be depressed in a study of 662 American mothers at 8 weeks (Dagher & Shenassa, 2012). Mothers of colicky babies had twice the rate of anxiety disorders compared to mothers of non-colicky babies in an Australian study of 232 mothers at 12 months (Christl et al., 2013). Thirty percent were depressed, 41% had high trait anxiety, 44% had past mental health problems, 38% had perfectionistic traits, and 32% had experienced past abuse. Some mothers were at higher risk, especially if they had unresolved issues around their own parenting, or if they had a trauma history.

That original hypothesis about infant crying and maternal depression is still correct, but it is much more complex than we originally believed. This chapter describes recent research on infant crying, temperament, sleep, and mother–infant bonding. Oddly, none of these studies include feeding method as a variable, but it is relevant to all the variables in this chapter. Since I described the role of feeding in Chapter 5, I will not describe it again here. But before I describe temperament, I want to suggest some physical reasons why babies cry so they can be addressed directly.

KEY FINDINGS

- Infant crying can increase mothers' risk of depression, but there are many factors that modify that relationship.
- Mothers who are depressed or have negative affect can increase infant fussiness.
- Prenatal depression can lead to epigenetic changes that increase infant fussiness.
- Depressed mothers' stress system overreacts when babies cry, suggesting that they, too, have experienced sensitization effects.
- Infant sleep often mediates the relationship between temperament and mothers' mental health. If babies do not sleep well and are fussy, their mothers are more likely to be depressed. (Keep in mind that breastfeeding would modify all these variables.)
- Male infants were more likely to have sleep issues and sensitive temperaments.
- Infant crying was associated with mothers' depressive symptoms and an insecure attachment.

DOI: 10.4324/9781003411246-24

Possible Physical Causes for Excessive Crying

Infants cry for many reasons. It is their only way to signal. They may be cold, bored, scared, or lonely, so carrying and babywearing often helps. Infants cry because they are hungry. Breastfeeding babies feed many times a day in the weeks as they are building their mothers' milk supply. Parents and others sometimes misunderstand this and think, "They *can't* be hungry—they *just ate*!" and so restrict their feeding. Babies may also be hungry if mothers report nipple pain or their weight is faltering. Tongue-tie, a condition where the baby's tongue is restricted by a tight frenulum, can also cause poor feeding, infant crying, and nipple pain and is frequently misdiagnosed (Kendall-Tackett, Walker, et al., 2018). A lactation consultant can rule out these problems.

Infants may cry because they were injured during birth and are uncomfortable. Infant chiropractic has reduced excessive crying in clinical trials (Miller, 2019, 2020). It may be something mothers would like to try. It usually works within a session or two. After ruling out physical causes for crying, we can consider the infant's temperament.

Infant Temperament

Babies with sensitive (or "difficult") temperaments have strong emotional reactions; cry for long periods of time; are hard to comfort; are slow to accept new people, foods, or routines; and may not sleep as well as babies with easier temperaments. Babies' interactions with their mothers or caregivers do not change temperament. It is hardwired. But interactions can modify it in negative or positive ways. Mothers' beliefs about their babies' temperament can increase their risk for depression—even more than how much babies objectively cry.

If a mother is confident, easygoing, and has support, her baby's temperament is unlikely to cause depression, even if the baby is fussy. Researchers describe this as synchrony, or "goodness of fit," between mother and baby. A study of 146 mothers from India found that 64% were confident, which had a positive influence on infant temperament (Jaya-Salengia et al., 2019). Family support increased mothers' confidence.

In contrast, mothers are more likely to be depressed if they describe their infants as difficult, even if they objectively are not. What mothers believe about their babies also influences how they respond to them. If mothers are inconsistent, angry, or intrusive, they can *cause* their infants to be fussy and unsettled. In one study, mothers' beliefs about their infants influenced infant affect regulation even more than maternal depression (Rosenblum et al., 2002). Mothers may resent their babies, as this mother describes.

> My first baby screamed from the day he was born. He screamed all the time, even in the hospital. He reacted oddly to all kinds of different things. The pediatrician said he was a "difficult" child. Even now, he has to have things always the same. . . . When I went back for a check-up at 2 weeks, a nurse asked me how the baby was. She said, "aren't they wonderful?" I didn't know what to say. I thought he was the pits.

Another mother had a fussy baby with little support. Her response was chilling and demonstrates why early intervention is so important.

> When the baby started throwing up, I felt terrible. I wouldn't go any place with her because I didn't want people to see her screaming. I wanted to be the perfect

mother. . . . My mother-in-law said, "you've got to relax. She's picking up on your cues. . . . The baby had a difficult temperament. Even now, she's very stubborn and strong-willed. . . . I wanted this baby so bad. When she came, I hated her. I thought of throwing her out the window. I just wanted her to die. I spanked her when she was 3 or 4 weeks old, and I'm still dealing with the guilt of it. . . . I'd yell at her, right in her face, "I hate you. I wish you would die."

Depressed mothers were more likely to say that their infants were difficult in a longitudinal study of 139 women at 8 months gestation, and at 2 and 6 months postpartum (McGrath et al., 2008). These differences were still apparent even after controlling for mothers' history of abuse or anxiety disorders. Depressed and non-depressed mothers reported equal levels of childcare stress and social support. The author recommended interventions that increased goodness of fit between mothers and babies.

Even among infants who were objectively colicky, a study from Sweden found that mothers' beliefs influenced their babies' symptoms (Canivet et al., 2002). Mothers who believed that too much contact would spoil a baby were more likely to have a colicky baby. Infants of these mothers were more distressed, even when given the same amount of physical contact as other babies.

The Effects of Prenatal Depression on Infant Temperament

Infant temperament is not as immutable as we once believed and can be shaped during pregnancy and early postpartum. Prenatal depression, anxiety, or PTSD appear to sensitize infants, making them fussier once they are born. For example, in a study of 253 pregnant women, infants of depressed mothers ($n = 83$) had signs of sensitization, including higher norepinephrine and cortisol (Field et al., 2007). These changes were associated with more sleep disturbances and less time in deep sleep.

If mothers were depressed during pregnancy/early postpartum, they were more likely to have babies with difficult temperaments at 6 months in a prospective study of 97 mother–infant dyads (Bang et al., 2020). Prenatal and postpartum depression also increased the number of colic episodes. Interestingly, these researchers also examined a traditional practice called *Taekyo*, where mothers were encouraged to think positively from early pregnancy to birth. *Taekyo* significantly increased prenatal attachment but did not lower risk for prenatal depression or depression at 6 to 8 weeks. However, mothers who practiced it were less depressed at 6 months.

Sensitization can also affect mothers' response to infant cries. Depressed pregnant women ($n = 22$) had a larger increase in systolic blood pressure than their non-depressed counterparts ($n = 50$) and were more sensitive to the sounds of infant distress (Pearson et al., 2012). Hypersensitivity to infant cries also increases the risk of abuse. In a study of 84 parents, 32 were considered high risk for physical abuse (Crouch et al., 2008). High- and low-risk parents watched a video of an infant crying. As predicted, high-risk parents rated the crying infant more negatively and had more hostile feelings after they watched the video than low-risk parents.

Temperament, Infant Sleep, and Maternal Mental Health

Babies with sensitive temperaments are notoriously poor sleepers, and infant sleep often mediates the relationship between infant temperament and mothers' mental health. A study measured depression at 2 to 4 days and 6 to 8 weeks postpartum in 204 women from Slovakia (Skodova et al., 2022). Depressed mothers were more likely to believe that their infants had sleeping problems and were sleeping a shorter amount of time than those of non-depressed mothers. (This may be more than belief. Prenatal depression may have objectively shortened infants' sleep time.) Frequency of night wakings was not related to depression. Infant temperament did not predict postpartum depression.

The Growing Up in New Zealand study (*n* = 5,568) measured prenatal depression, depression at 9 months, and infant sleep at 2 years (Kim et al., 2020). Prenatal depression increased risk of infant negative affect and toddler waking at 2 years. Prenatal depression, or prenatal and postpartum depression, doubled the risk of 2 or more night wakings, but postpartum depression alone did not. Maternal depression did not shorten infant sleep duration. Antenatal depression and increased night waking were related to two aspects of infant temperament: infant fear and negative affect, which suggest a sensitization effect. Prenatal depression directly increased night wakings and had an indirect effect on sleep via infant negative affect characteristics.

A study of 425 Canadian mothers found that mothers with postpartum major depression have substantially poorer sleep than their non-depressed counterparts at 4 to 8 weeks postpartum (Dennis & Ross, 2005). Mothers with pre-existing depression were excluded, so there were no in utero effects for infants. At 1 week, babies of depressed mothers cried more often and did not sleep well. Depressed mothers reported that their babies did not allow them to get a reasonable amount of sleep. These mothers woke three or more times a night and received less than 6 hours' sleep in a 24-hour period. Fussy babies slept less, and infant temperament mediated the relationship between infant sleep and maternal fatigue.

A study of 152 Israeli mothers at 5 to 8 months postpartum examined infant temperament and sleep, maternal mental health, and mother–infant bonding (Hairston et al., 2016). Eight percent of the women were depressed, but 67% reported infant sleep problems. Consistent with previous studies, infant sleep correlated with maternal mood and sleep. *Infant sleep problems were only a problem if the mothers were depressed.* Twenty-two percent of the variance in mother–infant bonding was explained by infant sleep problems and temperament. They suggested that cumulative maternal sleep loss due to infant sleep and feeding patterns explained maternal dysphoria.

A large population study from Norway (*n* = 86,724) found that depression at 6 months negatively impacted quality of life, but infant fussiness did not (Valla et al., 2022). One possible explanation for their finding is that by 6 months, fussiness had likely abated. Having a baby with normal sleep, feeling joy for having a baby, high relationship satisfaction were variables associated with quality of life.

Male Infants Are More Susceptible

Several studies have found that male infants are more susceptible to temperament and sleep issues. The ALSPAC study in the UK (*n* = 8,318) found that depression during pregnancy increased night waking at 8 months and shortened sleep duration at 24 months (Netsi et al., 2015). However, there was a three-way interaction effect: boys with more reactive temperaments and depressed mothers were the most susceptible to these effects.

A study of 64 full-term infants found altered sleep structure in infants of depressed mothers (Bat-Pitault et al., 2017). This included more awake time, a smaller percentage of non-rapid-eye-movement sleep (NREM), and less total sleep time. Male sex and reactive temperaments modified these effects. Mothers' expectations about infant sleep and the goodness of fit between the mother's and infant's temperament also modified this relationship.

In a study from Portugal, 164 mothers were assessed during their third trimester, and at 2 weeks and 3 and 6 months postpartum (Dias & Figueiredo, 2020). Prenatal depression increased infant sleep anxiety and daytime sleepiness. Mothers' depressive and anxiety symptoms at 2 weeks postpartum predicted more bedtime resistance and total sleep problems at 6 months. Consistent with previous studies, boys were more susceptible to these effects. Boys of mothers with prenatal depression had more sleep anxiety at 6 months.

Temperament, Sleep, Depression, and Mother–Infant Bonding

Temperament can also disrupt bonding via sleep problems and mothers' depression (Hairston et al., 2016). Crystal describes how her baby's fussiness interfered with her initial ability to bond with her baby. Once she identified a dairy allergy, her baby's symptoms improved, and she was able to attach to her baby.

> Kira [was] a fussy, unhappy baby. She would scratch at her face and pull her legs up to her stomach. . . . She would cry, spit up . . . none of this helped my bonding with her.
>
> Around 5 weeks postpartum, I cut dairy out of my diet. That . . . started to turn things around. . . . I cut out soy and nuts. . . . Friends and family encouraged me to wean, but no, this was something I could DO. . . .
>
> And over the following few weeks, the beautiful, happy little girl was allowed to come out, and I slowly felt able to bond with her.

In a prospective, longitudinal study, 22% of infants had colic symptoms, and 13% of mothers had major depression (Akman et al., 2008). Mothers of colicky babies were more depressed than mothers of non-colicky babies, and 63% of colicky infants were insecurely attached, compared with 31% of non-colicky infants. Infant colic was associated with both depressive symptoms and insecure attachment style.

Canadian researchers examined the relationship between infant health problems and crying at 12 months and mothers' psychosocial resources, such as secure adult attachments (Sawada et al., 2015). From a sample of 5,092 mothers, researchers identified 135 mothers who reported infant fussing and crying at 12 months or who had health problems at birth. Confirmatory factor analysis identified a variable called "felt security," which includes mothers' attachment, relationship quality, self-esteem, and social support. Infant health did not predict crying at 12 months, but the combination of mothers' prenatal felt security and infant health problems did.

A longitudinal study of 173 mother–infant dyads assessed mothers prenatally and up to 30 months (Newland et al., 2016). They examined goodness of fit, mother–infant sleep, and postpartum depression. Infant sleep patterns did not contribute to depression for all mothers, but mothers who required more sleep prenatally were affected by infant wakings at 15 months. At 30 months, mothers' prenatal sleep needs and infants' sleep indirectly affected mother–infant attachment.

Sleep- and temperament-related attachment issues can have long-ranging effects. In a prospective study of 64 infants referred for persistent crying, Wolke et al. (2002) compared them to a matched sample of 64 age mates. At 8 to 10 years, 19% of persistent criers had hyperactivity compared with 2% of control children. Parents of the persistent criers rated their children's temperaments as more negative, difficult, and demanding. Parents, and the children themselves, reported more conduct problems and lower academic achievement, especially for those with hyperactivity.

Clinical Takeaways

- If a baby is fussy, it is important to rule out physical causes before assuming that fussiness is due to temperament. Crying is the only way babies can communicate and often expresses a legitimate need. After ruling out feeding issues, chiropractic care is often helpful for excessive crying.
- Mothers of fussy babies need support and assistance to help them manage. Strategies, such as babywearing, can soothe fussiness. A support person can also give mothers a break so that they are not dealing with fussiness all by themselves.
- Treating mothers' depression can also help, as depressed mothers tend to view their infants more negatively and have a stronger physiologic response to crying.
- Holistic sleep coaching (not sleep training) can also help babies settle by considering the needs of both mother and baby, and developing strategies so that everyone can get more sleep.

18 Prematurity, Infant Illness, and Prior Infant Loss

Infants with health problems can also influence their mothers' emotional state. In addition, mothers' mental health can influence how they cope, how they see their children, and their level of attachment. Mothers with premature or ill infants need support, which can help prevent depression, anxiety, and PTSD.

KEY FINDINGS

- Mothers of preterm infants are at high risk for depression, anxiety, and PTSD. Mothers' symptoms are often related to their babies' illness. The sicker they are, the more likely mothers are to be depressed.
- ·Mothers and fathers of babies in the NICU are at high risk for acute stress disorder, the precursor to PTSD.
- Acute stress disorder (ASD) changed mothers' parenting behaviors because they could not help, hold, or care for their infants, protect them from pain, or share them with family members.
- Fathers had a delayed trauma response to babies in the NICU but may be even at higher risk.
- Mothers and fathers of very low-birthweight infants have PTSD that can last up to 5 years.
- Giving birth to a very low birthweight (VLBW) baby is a complex and ongoing trauma, not a single event.
- Kangaroo Mother Care and social support can help prevent depression and PTSD in mothers and fathers and increases mother–infant bonding.
- Mothers and fathers can have depression, anxiety, and PTSD following a stillbirth. These feelings may continue through a subsequent pregnancy.

Prematurity

Preterm birth can precipitate a psychological crisis. Mothers may experience guilt for an early delivery or anxiety or PTSD regarding the viability and morbidity of their infants. Preterm babies may also be born following a history of infertility, difficult pregnancy, or emergency delivery.

> My first child was premature. He was born at 35 weeks with severe Hyaline Membrane Disease. . . . He was in the hospital for five months. . . . The depression started around the time he was 3 or 4 weeks old. . . . Up until that time, everything had been so urgent. He had had a couple of arrests. It was overwhelming. Suddenly my son was doing better. Why was I feeling so bad? I had difficulties going to sleep

DOI: 10.4324/9781003411246-25

and was up several times during the night. It was difficult to wake up in the morning. I didn't want to do anything during the day except sleep and call the NICU to check in. I started not to eat well. I felt an impending sense of doom. The depression lasted about a month.

Mothers may also have a medical condition that precipitated an early delivery. This mother developed eclampsia, so her daughter was delivered 6 weeks premature via emergency cesarean section.

They took her away right after delivery. . . . They brought her back, but my arms were tied to the delivery table. I wish they had released at least one arm. . . . Leaving the hospital without the baby was really bad. I left early because I didn't want to leave at 11 a.m. with all the other moms and babies. . . . I shouldn't complain because she only had a few preemie problems. Others in the nursery were so sick. But it was very stressful. It was awful to see them putting the feeding tube down her throat, hearing her gagging and crying. It makes me cry now just to think about it.

Mothers often have delayed reactions to their babies' illness. They may be affected immediately, after a medical crisis, leaving the hospital without the baby, or once the baby is home. Sometimes, hospitals transfer babies who need specialized care. Mothers may find themselves alone in a strange city, cut off from their normal sources of support. These mothers are at particularly high risk.

When babies are critically ill, mothers may experience anticipatory grieving and begin·to mourn their loss. In this process, they may distance themselves from their babies to prepare for their eventual death. Infant recovery interrupts the mourning process, and mothers must readjust. Doctors told this mother that she had miscarried, only to find out that she was still pregnant. She experienced a similar type of grief and then struggled to reconnect.

My second pregnancy started off with tears. We went in for our first ultrasound and were told (and saw with our own eyes) that we had miscarried. The midwife showed where the gestational sac was breaking apart and there was nothing in it when we should have seen a heartbeat. We went home and cried, just waiting for the miscarriage to start. After a week of waiting and running to the bathroom every time I thought I felt any sort of discharge, we went back in for a follow-up ultrasound to see if I needed a D&C. Up on the screen popped a baby, and a heartbeat. The previous week, I had tried to emotionally separate myself from this baby. I found it hard to reconnect and be excited. The entire pregnancy I was plagued with the feeling that something was wrong.

Mothers of preterm infants often have frightening birth experiences and struggle with the care provided in the NICU. While many things have improved in NICU care, some providers are still insensitive, which can compound parents' fright, sadness, and anxiety. Providers may not acknowledge parents' feelings as they deal with a critically ill infant. Parents' reactions may surface months later, once their babies are out of danger, as this mother describes.

At 30 weeks pregnant, I started experiencing what I figured were Braxton Hicks contractions. We went to the hospital at the urging of my midwife because they were able to be timed at 5 minutes apart. The hospital confirmed I was in preterm labor. Since I was at the hospital my midwife did not have rights at, I was mainly seen by a resident whose bedside manner and wording of sensitive situations were lacking. . . .

After 4 days of labor, we couldn't stop it any longer and my little girl was born at 31 weeks. She was born by repeat c-section as our area hospitals don't allow VBAC. Since she was so ready to come out vaginally (they waited until the last possible minute), the surgeon had to pull on her neck and shoulders with more pressure than usual. He finally ended up doing a t-incision on my uterus, making future pregnancies extremely dangerous, to be able to pull her out. Minutes later, when I first saw her, her face was extremely purple from the bruising. The nurses said she looked like a domestic violence survivor.

The following 27 days in the NICU felt like a constant battle between what I knew was best for my daughter and not wanting to make the doctors mad, inevitably lengthening our stay. We battled with the required bottle feeding and needed supplementation, and not being allowed to nurse. . . .

After 27 days, she came home. My husband and I felt like zombies and were still so concerned about illness. We both showed signs (and still a year later, we both suffer) from what seems to be depression and PTSD.

Severity of Illness and Prematurity

The degree of illness or prematurity also influences maternal mental health. Some babies are hospitalized for only a few days, while others may be in intensive care for weeks or months. Whatever the circumstance, a preterm birth can increase the mother's risk of depression, anxiety, and PTSD.

Acute Stress Disorder (ASD) is the precursor syndrome to PTSD and does not require symptoms to be present for a month. Mothers and fathers with infants in the NICU are at high risk. A study from Boston Medical Center compared 59 low-income mothers with babies in the NICU to 60 similar mothers with well babies at 1 week postpartum (Vanderbilt et al., 2009). Thirty-nine percent of mothers with babies in the NICU were depressed compared with 22% of mothers of full-term babies. Twenty-four percent of NICU mothers met criteria for ASD compared with 3% of mothers of full-term babies.

Another study of 40 parents found that 44% of mothers of NICU babies met full criteria for acute stress disorder, while none of the fathers did (Shaw et al., 2006). Acute stress disorder changed parenting behavior. Mothers with ASD felt that they could not help, hold, or care for their infants, protect them from pain, or share them with other family members. Mothers' beliefs about their infants' illness better predicted their reactions than objective disease characteristics. Mothers with family support and a positive coping style were less likely to have trauma symptoms. The authors recommended involving parents more to make them feel less helpless, even with severely ill infants.

This same group of researchers extended their previous findings with a study of 18 parents (Shaw et al., 2009). At baseline, 55% of mothers met criteria for acute stress disorder, but none of the fathers. At 4 months, 33% of fathers, and 9% of mothers, met criteria for PTSD. Fathers had delayed trauma response but may be at even higher risk.

In a sample of 456 women from a high-risk maternity hospital in Rio de Janeiro, 9.4% of mothers met criteria for PTSD (Henriques et al., 2015). The risk factors for PTSD included 3 or more births, a 1-minute Apgar of 7 or less, history of mental health disorders, partner violence during pregnancy, unwanted sexual experience, and lifetime exposure to 5 or more traumas. Interestingly, none of the birth variables (birthweight, intrauterine growth retardation, fetal anomaly, or NICU admission) were related to PTSD, but mothers' lack of control and fear of birth predicted postpartum PTSD. Fifty-nine percent had cesareans, 20% were beaten while pregnant, and 12% reported psychological violence.

Very Low birthweight

Infants weighing 1,500 grams or below are considered very low birthweight (VLBW). These infants are more at risk for serious health complications, which increases their parents' risk for depression, anxiety, and PTSD. For example, 23% of mothers (*n* = 20) with very low birthweight babies in Quebec were in the clinical range for PTSD at 6 months corrected age (Feeley et al., 2011). Lower birthweight and more severe illness increased their mothers' PTSD symptoms. Severe PTSD symptoms decreased mothers' sensitivity as they interacted with their infants. Similarly, an American study compared 24 mothers of VLBW infants to 22 mothers of term infants at 2 to 3 years (Ahlund et al., 2009). Mothers of the VLBW infants had significantly more symptoms on all three trauma sub-scales (intrusion, avoidance, and hyperarousal) than mothers of term infants.

A series of German studies found having a VLBW infant negatively affects the mental health of mothers and fathers. The first study compared 50 mothers of VLBW infants to 30 control mothers (Kersting et al., 2004). Mothers of VLBW infants had more trauma symptoms, depression, and anxiety at all time points except 6 months, but none met full criteria for PTSD. Trauma symptoms did not diminish even at 14 months. The authors described giving birth to a VLBW baby as a complex and ongoing trauma, not a single event.

The second study included 230 mothers, and 173 fathers, and compared depression scores for parents of VLBW infant (*n* = 111) to parents of full-term infants (*n* = 119) at 4 to 6 weeks postpartum (Helle et al., 2015). Depression scores were 4 to 18 times higher in mothers of VLBW babies (depending on the measure), and 3 to 9 times higher in fathers. A 5-year longitudinal study included 250 families with either term or VLBW infants (Barkmann et al., 2018). As predicted, VLBW significantly predicted depression throughout the first 5 years for mothers and fathers. However, only 10% of mothers and fathers had severe depression.

Late Preterm Infants

Mothers can have difficulties even when their babies are only a few weeks early. These babies are called late preterm. One study compared 29 mothers of late preterm infants to 30 mothers whose babies were full-term (Brandon et al., 2011). Mothers of the late preterm infants had more depression and posttraumatic symptoms throughout the first month. Late preterm babies had more health problems and were in the hospital for a longer time, and their mothers worried more about their health. Their mothers had less time to prepare for the birth, and their babies had breastfeeding difficulties.

Infant Health and Behavior Problems

Infant health influences mothers' mental health, which influences how mothers interact with their infants. Social support influences this connection. A Swiss study compared 47 mothers of preterm infants to 25 mothers of full-term infants on mother–infant interaction style (Forcada-Guex et al., 2011). At 6 months corrected age, mothers of preterm infants with PTSD were more controlling in their interactions. The mothers of preterm infants without PTSD were more disengaged from their infants. Both styles led to poorer outcomes. In contrast, mothers of full-term infants were more likely to have a cooperative interaction style, which leads to better outcomes.

A sample of 102 predominantly Black and Hispanic mothers in the US examined the link between preterm birth, mother's depression, and infant's negative affect at 3 and 10 months (Barroso et al., 2015). These mothers had more preterm babies compared to normative samples. Using path analysis, low birthweight and preterm birth were directly related to postpartum depression, which predicted negative infant affect.

Low birthweight and prematurity also increased risk of health problems as children mature. A study of 27 preterm infants at 18 to 60 months found that children with a hyperreactive cortisol response had more attentional problems, anxiety, depression, and emotional reactivity than children in the sample without cortisol reactivity (Bagner et al., 2010). Children with high cortisol yelled, whined, and talked more negatively during a lab activity than children with low cortisol.

Another study conducted a cognitive assessment at 18 months and compared cortisol levels of three groups of infants: 25 infants at extremely low gestational age (ELGA: 24 to 28 weeks), 26 at very low gestation age (VLGA: 29 to 32 weeks), and 22 full-term (Brummelte et al., 2011). The ELGA infants had higher pretest cortisol, and their cortisol response pattern differed from the other two groups and increased the risk of dysfunctional mother–infant interactions. Encouragingly, if mothers of preterm infants used a positive interaction style, it lowered cortisol. This was not true for full-term infants. The authors hypothesized that the HPA axis changed in response to extreme prematurity.

Kangaroo Mother Care

Kangaroo Mother Care is a useful technique for parents of premature infants. It involves placing the baby, wearing only a diaper, between the mother's breasts, with babies in a sling or pouch. (This also works well with partners and other family members.) Babies benefit almost immediately. They are calmer, and their body temperature stabilizes. They cry less, which conserves calories and allows them to grow. They are discharged from the hospital earlier. Mothers also feel more confident, breastfeeding is established, and their babies are more likely to form secure attachments.

Parmar and colleagues (2009) studied families of 135 babies from India with an average birthweight of 1460 grams and a gestational age of 30 weeks. Kangaroo mother care (KMC) started in the first week of life. KMC improved oxygen saturation level, temperature and respiration stabilized, and heart rate lowered by 3 to 5 beats. Ninety-six percent of the mothers, 82% of the fathers, and 84% of other family members accepted Kangaroo Mother Care as a treatment. Mothers felt closer to their babies and reported that KMC elevated their mood, although they were initially frightened about trying it. Mothers felt more confident in handling their babies. Healthcare workers also reported that mothers feel more confident and it increased breastfeeding. Babies also cried less and slept more.

Kangaroo Mother Care also specifically helps with postpartum depression. In a randomized trial of Kangaroo Mother Care for mothers of low-birthweight infants in Northern India, 974 mothers were in the intervention group, and 852 in the control group

(Sinha et al., 2021). The overall rate of moderate to severe postpartum depression was 10.8% for the intervention group vs 13.6% for the control group. There was no difference in day 28 cortisol levels or breastfeeding, but the authors noted that for every 36 mothers who do Kangaroo Mother Care, 1 mother would be prevented from having moderate to severe depression, which they considered a substantial reduction in risk.

In a case study, Dombrowski and colleagues (2001) found that Kangaroo Mother Care helped a mother at very high risk for depression. She was 22 years old, single, and had given up a previous baby for adoption. She and her younger brother were removed from their home when she was 5 because of her father's repeated physical and sexual abuse. She and her brother were adopted at age 9, after four years in multiple foster homes. The mother had an active history of substance use. Her baby was premature, and she was severely depressed. However, within 24 hours of starting Kangaroo Mother Care, she was no longer depressed. She was assessed at 6 weeks, 3 months, and 7 months and was neither depressed nor using substances. She described her experience as follows:

> It was important to both of us for bonding. It made me feel closer than I felt holding her regular, you know, wrapped. It calmed her down a lot more and made her more secure. It made me close to her and I was scared to be a mother, but it gave me a sense of peace that I could do it (take care of the baby). It made me less stressed and able to relax—a "time out" together kind of thing. I was able to forget everything else. It worked well for both of us on stress. I felt like I needed something and being a recovering drug addict, I needed this to help.
>
> (p. 215)

Kangaroo Mother Care also helped full-term babies in a randomized trial that included 100 healthy neonates from Iran (Kashaninia et al., 2008). The infants in the Kangaroo Mother Care group were held 10 minutes before and during an injection. The Kangaroo Mother Care infants had a significantly lower scores on the Neonatal Infant Pain Scale than infants in the control group and cried for a shorter amount of time.

Social Support Intervention

Another intervention has also improved outcomes for mothers of premature babies (Jotzo & Poets, 2005). In this study, mothers were randomly assigned to a crisis intervention 5 days after birth, or they received usual care. The intervention took place in the NICU two times a week, for 5 to 15 minutes. The crisis intervention included helping mothers reconstruct the events before and after their births, teaching them relaxation techniques, explaining stress and trauma responses, providing them with support during "emotional outbursts," discussing with them personal resources and current support, and offering them possible solutions for concrete problems. At discharge, mothers in the intervention group had significantly lower trauma symptoms than mothers who received standard care.

A more recent study from Iran trained fathers of NICU infants to provide social support for their wives. The study compared 30 mothers in an intervention group to 45 mothers in a usual-care group (Shirazi et al., 2022). The intervention was two 90-minute sessions designed to teach fathers of preterm babies how to support their wives with techniques such as skin-to-skin contact, infant massage, and infant feeding. This simple intervention lowered mothers' stress and increased their self-efficacy compared with mothers in the usual-care group.

Assisted Reproductive Technologies and Prior Infant Loss

Mothers may also have a history of infertility, miscarriage, or fetal loss, which increases their risk for depression and anxiety for subsequent pregnancies. Italian researchers compared a sample of 48 parents who used assisted reproductive technology (ART; 25 mothers, 23 fathers) with 39 non-ART mothers at 30 to 32 weeks' gestation, and at 1 week and 3 months postpartum (Monti et al., 2009). ART mothers were more depressed at all assessment points than non-ART women, with depression at its highest rate during pregnancy. Interestingly, the men in ART couples were not depressed at the first two assessment points but were at 3 months.

A recent study of 1,789 new mothers from Northern Uganda included 77 mothers who had experienced stillbirths or early neonatal deaths (Arach et al., 2020). The perinatal death rate in Uganda is high: 40 per 1,000 births, with 33% living in poverty. In the total sample, 21% of mothers were depressed. Recent perinatal loss increased the risk of depression by 3.45 times.

Prior infant loss increased the risk for PTSD, depression, and anxiety with a subsequent birth in a sample of 36 mothers and fathers (Armstrong et al., 2009). While depression and anxiety decreased over time, PTSD remained in the moderately high range throughout pregnancy and increased from the third trimester to 6 to 8 months postpartum. Mothers and fathers had similar rates of posttraumatic stress symptoms.

In a review of 17 studies, Badenhorst et al. (2006) found that fathers grieved but had less guilt than mothers. They had anxiety, depression, and PTSD, but at lower levels than mothers. They concluded that fathers also need help before they can support their partners.

A descriptive phenomenological study of 12 mothers explored mothers' and fathers' experiences of ultrasound following infant loss in the previous year (O'Leary, 2005). Many learned that their first babies had died during a previous ultrasound. Current ultrasound reminded them of that prior event: the smells, sights, feelings, and sounds of the ultrasound room. During the ultrasound, some mothers experienced flashbacks to their previous loss—even when the current baby was healthy. Both fathers and mothers showed equal levels of trauma following the ultrasound. Based on her research, O'Leary (2005) recommended preparing parents for possible flashbacks during ultrasound. Let them hear the heartbeat first before the ultrasound. Acknowledge and validate the parents' concerns while assuring them that the current baby is healthy. Finally, recognize that fathers may be as traumatized as mothers.

Karin describes her experience with her stillbirth and subsequent high-risk pregnancy and preterm birth. Her baby was in the NICU for 13 days. She eventually developed postpartum OCD at 6 months postpartum.

> After a traumatic stillbirth at 19 weeks, I found myself immediately pregnant with baby number 2. . . .
> My doctor recommended a procedure to ensure a healthy delivery at a better time for our son: a cerclage. . . . When the 2 weeks had passed after the cerclage, I went back to work part-time. I ended up in preterm labor and it was stopped with drugs. I had to quit my job and begin complete bedrest.

For 17 weeks, I laid in my bed and hoped my baby would stay in for one more day. I obsessed about how far along I was, if I had felt my baby move recently, and how many contractions I was having. The thought that I would have to bury another baby was exhausting.

. . . At 33 weeks, I started experiencing back labor, so my OB/Gyn gave me a dose of betamethasone. . . . The next day, the contractions continued, and . . . I had an infection. . . . A cesarean delivery was prepared. As soon as my husband walked in, they dressed him in scrubs and rolled me back to the OR.

While Zeke had a high 1-minute APGAR, he started struggling almost immediately after that. He was intubated and taken to the NICU. I first saw him as I was wheeled past his isolette after surgery.

. . . The NICU staff allowed my husband to be the first to hold him. Even 16 years later, I am angry at the staff for knowing that was an important time, and not waiting for me. I was so young (21). I didn't know how to be an advocate for myself or my son. . . .

He was called a "feeder/grower," and even though we didn't have to worry too much about future problems, the constant vigilance to the monitors and mLs of milk was exhausting. . . . We took him home on preemie formula fortification on my milk, with very little instruction. It felt like we were being tossed to the wind. We had never done his daily care for longer than an hour at a time. The experts had done it. We felt so alone and unprepared for taking this tiny human home.

A US survey of 769 mothers who had had a stillbirth in the past 18 months found that family support lowered the risk of anxiety and depression (Cacciatore et al., 2009). While mothers noted that support from nurses, physicians, and groups was helpful, only family support had a significant effect on anxiety and depression.

This mother lost her first son when he was born at 24 weeks. Her second pregnancy was difficult and ended with an emergency cesarean. She felt disconnected and in a daze for the first 7 months of her baby's life.

In 2008, I lost my first baby . . . after two hours because his lungs were not developed enough for him to survive. I struggled with a deep grief after that, the very worst feelings I have ever experienced in my life.

When I became pregnant again . . . my pregnancy was filled with anxiety, constant ultrasounds, bed rest and worry. When I went into labor at 41 weeks, I was so excited and proud to have reached that point. My labor progressed and seemed to be going well until my OB called a code red, cord prolapse, everything turned to panic as I was rushed to the ER having to leave my husband behind. I remember stopping the nurse before I passed out, asking her to tell me if my baby was OK, and her answer was "we can't tell you that."

Thankfully, my son, Darragh, was perfect, but I spent the next few months in a daze. When he was 7 months old, I finally asked my doctor for help. I felt out of control, panicked, and so isolated. She sent me to a psychologist, and I was prescribed Celexa. I had never done the "drugs" thing before and felt like a failure. But it helped so much. A cloud and weight were lifted.

I have had another two boys since, I'm still on Celexa and have not had any significant PPD.

A study compared 62 women who had late-term terminations for fetal anomalies, 43 mothers who had very low-birthweight babies, and 65 mothers with healthy infants (Kersting et al., 2009). At 14 days, 22% of mothers in the termination group had psychiatric disorders (PTSD, depression, and anxiety), compared with 19% of mothers of very low-birthweight infants, and 6% of mothers with full-term infants. At 14 months, the rates for the mothers in the termination group were 17%, and preterm-infant group 7%. None of the mothers of full-term infants had psychiatric conditions at 14 months. The authors concluded that both late terminations and giving birth to a very preterm baby can cause substantial psychological distress, even up to 14 months later.

Clinical Takeaways

- Mothers and at-risk babies bring special challenges to their relationship. Mothers may be in the process of grieving when they are forced to deal with babies who are different from what they expected and may be difficult to handle.
- Despite these difficulties, attachment can develop between mother and baby, especially if the mother is adequately supported and she perceives it as support.
- You can do much to facilitate these types of positive reactions. Helping mothers feel competent in caring for their babies is vital for reducing risk for postpartum depression and facilitating a secure attachment.

Epilogue
Some Final Thoughts

There is much you can do to help new mothers who have postpartum depression, anxiety, or PTSD. Here are some final thoughts to send you on your way.

Listen to Mothers

Just letting a mother tell her story can be therapeutic. Sometimes mothers know and can articulate what is bothering them. They just need someone to hear and validate their concerns. If we listen and the mother feels we've truly heard her, she'll be more likely to follow our suggestions.

Let Mothers Know about Factors That Might Be Influencing Their Emotional State

After listening carefully, then it is time to share what you know. Sometimes mothers really do not know why they feel bad. This can be true even years later. Dozens of times, I've been teaching a seminar and had participants come up and say that they never realized that a crying baby (or some other factor they identified with) could have caused their emotional distress. These women are generally healthcare providers with grown children. Having someone simply name the factors involved can validate mothers and let them know that they are not alone.

Offer Specific Suggestions That Can Help

Once you have narrowed down some possible causes, offer her some strategies to help address the problems. For example, if she is having nipple pain, address the problem or refer her to a lactation specialist. If a mother is highly fatigued, brainstorm with her about how she can get more rest, and help her mobilize her support network. Also, be sure to rule out physical problems. If she has a baby with a difficult temperament or was premature, put her in contact with other mothers you know who have similar issues, and teach her some strategies to cope with babies who might not settle easily.

Help Her Mobilize Her Own Support System, Including Offering Referrals to People or Organizations That Can Offer Long-Term Support

Your role is pivotal in terms of helping mothers identify depression, anxiety, and PTSD and referring them to the sources of help. It is not practical (usually) for you to be a

DOI: 10.4324/9781003411246-26

mother's long-term source of support. You can help mothers find support among their own network and in their own communities.

One helpful thing you can do is give mothers "permission" to get help and support. So often, mothers believe that they must tough things out. Over the years, I've had many mothers repeat the apocryphal tale of the mother in the field who gives birth and gets right back to work. Yes, unfortunately, this does happen—especially in impoverished communities. But it is far from ideal and, as I described in Chapter 16, is not the norm. Nor is it something to aspire to. I have found it helpful to describe what happens in cultures that support new mothers and reiterate that support is the goal.

You might also have to refer mothers for other types of help. Resources can include support groups on various topics (breastfeeding, depression, difficult birth, premature babies, childbearing loss, mothering multiples, or single mothering). In rural communities, websites and Facebook groups can be very helpful. Mothers may also need referrals for therapy and/or medications. Organizations such as Postpartum Support International (www.postpartum.net) provide referral lists and now offer telehealth appointments. They also have a US hotline staffed 24/7.

If you are not a mental health provider, your state and province psychological associations also provide referrals for professionals in your community who can help depressed mothers. I recommend that you speak with these individuals before referring mothers, however. Also, be sure to find out what their payment policy is—especially for your low-income mothers.

Conclusions

I have long believed that prompt intervention can stop the downward spiral of postpartum mental illness and prevent so much suffering. In closing, I'd like to share the words of Salle Webber, a postpartum doula who understands the pivotal role you can have in young families.

> Incredible as it seems, our culture, with its emphasis on education, has left young adults entirely unprepared to face the practical realities of parenting. And this may be the most important job they will ever hold. So, for those of us who are comfortable and happy in the work of parenting, we can serve the future of humanity through our humble sharing of our skills and our love for children and families.
> (Webber, 1992, p. 17)

I wish you great success in this important work.

References

Abramowitz, J. S., Meltzer-Brody, S., Leserman, J., Killenberg, S., Rinaldi, K., Mahaffey, B. L., & Pedersen, C. (2010). Obsessional thoughts and compulsive behaviors in a sample of women with postpartum mood symptoms. *Archives of Women's Mental Health*, *13*, 523–530. https://doi.org/10.1007/s00737-010-0172-4

Abramowitz, J. S., Schwartz, S. A., Moore, K., & Luenzmann, K. R. (2003). Obsessive-compulsive symptoms in pregnancy and the puerperium: A review of the literature. *Journal of Anxiety Disorders*, *17*(4), 461–478. https://doi.org/0.1016/s0887-6185(02)00206-2

Adewuya, A. O., Ologun, Y. A., & Ibigbami, O. S. (2006). Post-traumatic stress disorder after childbirth in Nigerian women: Prevalence and risk factors. *British Journal of Obstetrics & Gynecology*, *113*, 284–288.

Adeyemo, E. O., Oluwole, E. O., Kanma-Okafor, O. J., Izuka, O. M., & Odeyemi, K. A. (2020). Prevalence and predictors of postpartum depression among postnatal women in Lagos, Nigeria. *African Health Sciences*, *20*(4), 1943–1954. https://doi.org/https://dx.doi.org/10.4314/ahs

Ahlqvist-Bjorkroth, S., Vaarno, J., Junttila, N., Pajulo, M., Raiha, H., Niinikoski, H., & Lagstrom, H. (2016). Initiation and exclusivity of breastfeeding: Association with mothers' and fathers' prenatal and postnatal depression and marital distress. *Acta Obstetrica Gynecologica Scandanavica*, *95*(4), 396–404. https://doi.org/10.1111/aogs.12857

Ahlund, S., Clarke, P., Hill, J., & Thalange, N. K. S. (2009). Post-traumatic stress symptoms in mothers of very low birth weight infants 2–3 years postpartum. *Archives of Women's Mental Health*, *12*, 261–264.

Ahmed, A., Stewart, D. E., Teng, L., Wahoush, O., & Gagnon, A. J. (2008). Experience of immigrant new mothers with symptoms of depression. *Archives of Women's Mental Health*, *11*(4), 295–303.

Ahn, S., & Corwin, E. J. (2015). The association between breastfeeding, the stress response, inflammation, and postpartum depression during the postpartum period: Prospective cohort study. *International Journal of Nursing Studies*, *52*, 1582–1590.

Ahokas, A., Aito, M., & Rimon, R. (2000). Positive treatment effect of estradiol in postpartum psychosis: A pilot study. *Journal of Clinical Psychiatry*, *61*, 166–169.

Ahokas, A., Kaukoranta, J., Wahlbeck, K., & Aito, M. (2001). Estrogen deficiency in severe postpartum depression: Successful treatment with sublingual physiologic 17-beta estradiol: A preliminary study. *Journal of Clinical Psychiatry*, *62*, 332–336.

Akman, I., Kuscu, K., Ozdemir, N., Yurdakul, Z., Solakoglu, M., Orhan, L., & Karabekiroglu, A. (2008). Mothers' postpartum psychological adjustment and infantile colic. *Archives of Diseases of Childhood*, *91*, 417–419.

Alcorn, K. L., O'Donovan, A., Patrick, J. C., Creedy, D., & Devilly, G. J. (2010). A prospective longitudinal study of the prevalence of post-traumatic stress disorder resulting from childbirth events. *Psychological Medicine*, *40*, 1849–1859.

Alvarez-Segura, M., Garcia-Esteve, L., Torres, A., Plaza, A., Imaz, M. L., Hermida-Barros, L., San, L., & Burtchen, N. (2014). Are women with a history of abuse more vulnerable to perinatal depressive symptoms? A systematic review. *Archives of Women's Mental Health*, *17*, 343–357.

American Psychiatric Association. (2022). *Diagnostic and statistical manual* (5th ed., Text Rev.). DSM-5-TR. `American Psychiatric Association.

Anda, R. F., Brown, D. W., Felitti, V. J., Bremner, J. D., Dube, S. R., & Giles, W. H. (2007). Adverse childhood experiences and prescribed psychotropic medications in adults. *American Journal of Preventive Medicine*, *32*(5), 389–394. https://doi.org/S0749-3797(07)00011-6 [pii] 10.1016/j.amepre.2007.01.005

Anda, R. F., Croft, J. B., Felitti, V. J., Nordenberg, D., Giles, W. H., Williamson, D. F., & Giovino, G. (1999). Adverse childhood experiences and smoking during adolescence and adulthood. *Journal of the American Medical Association*, *282*, 1652–1658.

Anda, R. F., Dong, M., Brown, D. W., Felitti, V. J., Giles, W. H., Perry, G. S., Valerie, E. J., & Dube, S. R. (2009). The relationship of adverse childhood experiences to a history of premature death of family members. *BMC Public Health*, *9*, 106. https://doi.org/1471-2458-9-106 [pii] 10.1186/1471-2458-9-106

Anderson, L. N., Campbell, M. K., daSilva, O., Freeman, T., & Xie, B. (2008). Effect of maternal depression and anxiety on use of health services for infants. *Canadian Family Physician*, *54*, e1711–1715, e1718–e1719.

Ansara, D., Cohen, M. M., Gallop, R., Kung, R., Kung, R., & Schei, B. (2005). Predictors of women's physical health problems after childbirth. *Journal of Psychosomatic Obstetrics & Gynecology*, *26*, 115–125.

Arach, A. A. O., Nakajujja, N., Nankabirwa, V., Ndeezi, G., Kiguli, J., Mukunya, D., Odongkara, B., Achora, V., Tongun, J. B., WMusaba, M. W., Napyo, A., Zalwango, V., Tylleskar, T., & Tumwine, J. K. (2020). Perinatal death triples the prevalence of postpartum depression among women in Northern Uganda: A community-based cross-sectional study. *PLoS One*, *15*(10), e0240409. https://doi.org/https://doi.org/10.1371/journal.pone.0240409

Armstrong, D. S., Hutti, M. H., & Myers, J. (2009). Parents' psychological distress after the birth of a subsequent healthy infant. *Journal of Obstetric, Gynecologic, and Neonatal Nursing*, *38*, 654–666.

Arnold, M., & Kalibatseva, Z. (2021). Are "superwomen" without social support at risk for postpartum depression and anxiety? *Women & Health*, *61*(2), 148–159. https://doi.org/https://doi.org/10.1080/03630242.2020.1844360

Aronsson, C. A., Lee, H.-S., Liu, E., Uusitalo, U., Hummel, S., Yang, J., Hummel, M., Rewers, M., She, J.-X., Simell, O., Toppari, J., Ziegeler, A.-G., Krischer, J., Virtanen, S. M., Norris, J. M., Agardh, D., & The TEDDY Study Group. (2015). Age at gluten introduction and risk of celiac disease. *Pediatrics*, *135*(2), 239–245. https://doi.org/10.1542/peds.2014-1787

Asper, M. M., Hallen, N., Lindberg, L., Mansdotter, A., Carlberg, M., & Wells, M. B. (2018). Screening fathers for postpartum depression can be cost-effective: An example from Sweden. *Journal of Affective Disorders*, *241*, 154–163. https://doi.org/https://doi.org/10.1016/j.jad.2018.07.044

Aswathi, A., Rajendiren, S., Nimesh, A., Philip, R. R., Kattimani, S., Jayalakshmi, D., Ananthanarayanan, P. H., & Dhiman, P. (2015). High serum testosterone levels during the postpartum period are associated with postpartum depression. *Asian Journal of Psychiatry*, *17*, 85–88.

Ayers, S., Bond, R., Bertullies, S., & Wijma, K. (2016). The aetiology of posttraumatic stress following childbirth: A meta-analysis and theoretical framework. *Psychological Medicine*, *46*(6), 1121–1134. https://doi.org/10.1017/S0033291715002706

Ayers, S., Eagle, A., & Waring, H. (2006). The effects of childbirth-related post-traumatic stress disorder on women and their relationships: A qualitative study. *Psychology, Health & Medicine*, *11*(4), 389–398.

Ayers, S., Harris, R., Sawyer, A., Parfitt, Y., & Ford, E. (2009). Posttraumatic stress disorder after childbirth: Analysis of symptom presentation and sampling. *Journal of Affective Disorders, 119,* 200–204.

Badenhorst, W., Riches, S., Turton, P., & Hughes, P. (2006). The psychological effects of stillbirth and neonatal death on fathers: Systematic review. *Journal of Psychosomatic Obstetrics & Gynecology, 27*(4), 245–256.

Bagner, D. M., Sheinkopf, S. J., Vohr, B. R., & Lester, B. M. (2010). A preliminary study of cortisol reactivity and behavior problems in young children born premature. *Developmental Psychobiology, 52*(6), 574–582.

Bandelow, B., Sojka, F., Broocks, A., Hajak, G., Bleich, S., & Ruther, E. (2006). Panic disorder during pregnancy and the postpartum period. *European Psychiatry, 21,* 495–500.

Bang, K.-S., Lee, I., Kim, S., Yi, Y., Huh, I., Jang, S.-Y., Kim, D., & Lee, S. (2020). Relation between mother's Taekyo, prenatal and postpartum depression, and infant's temperament and colic: A longitudinal prospective approach. *International Journal of Environmental Research and Public Health, 17,* 7691. https://doi.org/10.3390/ijerph17207691

Barber, G. A., & Shenassa, E. D. (2021). Smoking status: A tacit screen for postpartum depression in primary care settings. *Journal of Affective Disorders, 295,* 1243–1250. https://doi.org/https://doi.org/10.1016/j.jad.2021.09.033

Barkmann, C., Helle, N., & Bindt, C. (2018). Is very low birthweight a predictor for a five-year course of depression in parents? A latent growth curve model. *Journal of Affective Disorders, 229,* 415–420.

Barooj-Kiakalaee, O., Hosseini, S.-H., Mohammad-Tahmtan, R.-A., Hosseini-Tabaghdehi, M., Jahanfar, S., Esmaeili-Douki, Z., & Shahhosseini, Z. (2022). Paternal postpartum depression's relationship to maternal pre and postpartum depression, and father-mother dyads marital satisfaction: A structural equation model analysis of a longitudinal study. *Journal of Affective Disorders, 297,* 375–380. https://doi.org/https://doi.org/10.1016/j.jad.2021.10.110

Barr, J. A., & Beck, C. T. (2008). Infanticide secrets: Qualitative study on postpartum depression. *Canadian Family Physician, 54,* e1716–e1717, e1711–e1715.

Barrios, Y. V., Gelaye, B., Zhong, Q., Nicolaidis, C., Rondon, M. B., Garcia, P. J., Sanchez, P. A., Sanchez, S. E., & Williams, M. A. (2015). Association of childhood physical and sexual abuse with intimate partner violence, poor general health, and depressive symptoms. *PLoS One.* https://doi.org/10.1371/journal.pone.0116609

Barroso, N. E., Hartley, C. M., Bagner, D. M., & Pettit, J. W. (2015). The effect of preterm birth on infant negative affect and maternal postpartum depressive symptoms: A preliminary examination in an underrepresented minority sample. *Infant Behavior & Development, 39,* 159–165.

Barry, T. J., Murray, L., Pasco Fearon, R. M., Moutsiana, C., Cooper, P. J., Goodyer, J. M., Herbert, J., & Halligan, S. L. (2015). Maternal postnatal depression predicts altered offspring biological stress reactivity in adulthood. *Psychoneuroendocrinology, 52,* 251–260.

Bascom, E. M., & Napolitano, M. A. (2016). Breastfeeding duration and primary reasons for breastfeeding cessation among women with postpartum depressive symptoms. *Journal of Human Lactation, 32*(2), 282–291.

Basu, A., Kim, H. H., Basaldua, R., Choi, K. W., Charron, L., Kelsall, N., Hernandez-Diaz, S., Wyszynski, D. F., & Koenen, K. C. (2021). A cross-national study of factors associated with women's perinatal mental health and wellbeing during the COVID-19 pandemic. *PLoS One, 16*(4). https://doi.org/https://doi.org/10.1371/journal.pone.0249780

Bat-Pitault, F., Sesson, G., Deruelle, C., Flori, S., Porcher-Guinet, V., Stagnara, C., Guyon, A., Plancoulaine, S., Adrien, J., Da Fonseca, D., Patural, H., & Franco, P. (2017). Altered sleep architecture during the first months of life in infants born to depressed mothers. *Sleep Medicine, 30,* 195–203.

Bauman, B. L., Ko, J. Y., Cox, S., D'Angelo, D. V., Warner, L., Folger, S., Tevendale, H. D., Coy, K. C., Harrison, L., & Barfield, W. D. (2020). Postpartum depressive symptoms and provider discussions about perinatal depression: United States 2018. *Morbidity & Mortality Weekly Report*, 69(19), 575–581.

Baumeister, D., Akhtar, R., Pariante, C. M., & Mondelli, V. (2016). Childhood trauma and adult-hood inflammation: A meta-analysis of peripheral C-reactive protein, interleukin-6, and tumour necrosis factor-alpha. *Molecular Biology*, 21(5), 642–649. https://doi.org/10.1038/mp.2015.67

Beck, C. T. (2002). Postpartum depression: A meta-analysis. *Qualitative Health Research*, 12, 453–472.

Beck, C. T. (2006). Postpartum depression: It isn't just the blues. *American Journal of Nursing*, 106(5), 40–50.

Beck, C. T. (2009). An adult survivor of child sexual abuse and her breastfeeding experience: A case study. *MCN American Journal of Maternal Child Nursing*, 34(2), 91–97.

Beck, C. T. (2011). A meta-ethnography of traumatic childbirth and its aftermath: Amplifying causal looping. *Qualitative Health Research*, 21. https://doi.org/10.1177/1049732310390698

Beck, C. T. (2015). Middle range theory of traumatic childbirth: The ever-widening ripple effect. *Global Qualitative Nursing Research*. https://doi.org/10.1177/23333393615575313

Beck, C. T., Gable, R. K., Sakala, C., & Declercq, E. R. (2011). Posttraumatic stress disorder in new mothers: Results from a two-stage U.S. national survey. *Birth*, 38(3), 216–227.

Beck, C. T., & Watson, S. (2008). Impact of birth trauma on breast-feeding. *Nursing Research*, 57(4), 228–236.

Bei, B., Milgrom, J., Ericksen, J., & Trinder, J. (2010). Subjective perception of sleep, but not its objective quality, is associated with immediate postpartum mood disturbances in healthy women. *Sleep*, 33(4), 531–538.

Berglink, V., Gibney, S. M., & Drexhage, H. A. (2014). Autoimmunity, inflammation, and psy-chosis: A search for peripheral markers. *Biological Psychiatry*, 75(4), 324–331. doi: 10.1016/j.biopsych.2013.09.037.

Berman, H., Mason, R., Hall, J., Rodger, S., Classen, C. C., Evans, M. K., Ross, L. E., Mulcahy, G. A., Carranza, L., & Al-Zoubi, F. (2014). Laboring to mother in the context of past trauma: The transition to motherhood. *Qualitative Health Research*, 24, 1253–1264. https://doi.org/10.1177/1049732314521902

Bhatti, S., & Richards, K. (2015). A systematic review of the relationship between postpartum sleep disturbance and postpartum depression. *Journal of Obstetric, Gynecologic, and Neonatal Nursing*, 44(3), 350–357. https://doi.org/10.1111/1552-6909.12562

Black, K. A., MacDonald, I., Chambers, T., & Ospina, M. B. (2019). Postpartum mental health disorders in Indigenous women: A systematic review and meta-analysis. *Journal of Obstet-rics & Gynaecology Canada*, 41(10), 1470–1479. https://doi.org/https://doi.org/10.1016/j.jogc.2019.02.009

Bloch, M., Schmidt, P. J., Danaceau, M., Murphy, J., Niemann, L., & Rubinow, D. R. (2000). Effects of gonadal steroids in women with a history of postpartum depression. *American Journal of Psychiatry*, 157, 924–930.

Borra, C., Iacovou, M., & Sevilla, A. (2015). New evidence on breastfeeding and postpartum depression: The importance of understanding women's intentions. *Maternal & Child Health Journal*, 19(4), 897–907.

Boufidou, F., Lambrinoudaki, I., Argeitis, J., Zervas, I. M., Pliatsika, P., Leonardou, A. A., Petro-poulos, G., Hasiakos, D., Papadias, K., & Nikolaou, C. (2009). CSF and plasma cytokines at delivery and postpartum mood disorders. *Journal of Affective Disorders*, 115, 287–292.

Brand, S. R., Engel, S. M., Canfield, R. L., & Yehuda, R. (2006). The effect of maternal PTSD following in utero trauma exposure on behavior and temperament in the 9-month-old infant. *Annals of the New York Academy of Sciences*, 1071, 454–458.

Brandon, D. H., Tully, K. P., Silva, S. G., Malcolm, W. F., Murtha, A. P., & Turner, B. S. (2011). Emotional responses of mothers of late-preterm and term infants. *Journal of Obstetric, Gyneco-logic, and Neonatal Nursing*, 40, 719–731.

Brummelte, S., & Galea, L. A. M. (2016). Postpartum depression: Etiology, treatment, and conse-quences for maternal care. *Hormones & Behavior*, 77, 153–166.

Brummelte, S., Grunau, R. E., Zaidman-Zait, A., Weinberg, J., Nordstokke, D., & Cepeda, I. L. (2011). Cortisol levels in relation to maternal interaction and child internalizing behavior in preterm and full-term children at 18 month corrected age. *Developmental Psychobiology, 53*(2), 184–195.

Bryson, H., Perlen, S., Price, A., Mensah, F., Gold, L., Dakin, P., & Goldfeld, S. (2021). Patterns of maternal depression, anxiety, and stress symptoms from pregnancy to 5 years postpartum in an Australian cohort experiencing adversity. *Archives of Disease of Childhood, 24*, 987–997. https://doi.org/https://doi.org/10.1007/s00737-021-01145-0

Buemann, B., Marazziti, D., & Uvnas-Moberg, K. (2021). Can intravenous oxytocin infusion counteract hyperinflammation in COVID-19 infected patients? *World Journal of Biological Psychiatry, 22*(5), 387–398. https://doi.org/10.1080/15622975.2020.1814408

Bugental, D. B., Beaulieu, D., & Schwartz, A. (2008). Hormonal sensitivity of preterm versus full-term infants to the effects of maternal depression. *Infant Behavior & Development, 31*, 51–61.

Buss, C., Davis, E. P., Shahbaba, B., Pruessner, J. C., Head, K., & Sandman, C. A. (2012). Maternal cortisol over the course of pregnancy and subsequent child amygdala and hippocampus volumes and affective problems. *Proceedings of the National Academy of Sciences USA, 109*(20), E1312–E1319.

Buttner, M. M., Mott, S. L., Pearlstein, T., Stuart, S., Zlotnick, C., & O'Hara, M. W. (2013). Examination of premenstrual symptoms as a risk factor for depression in postpartum women. *Archives of Women's Mental Health, 16*, 219–225.

Cabizuca, M., Marques-Portella, C., Mendlowicz, M. V., Coutinho, E. S. F., & Figueira, I. (2009). Posttraumatic stress disorder in parents of children with chronic illnesses: A meta-analysis. *Health Psychology, 28*(3), 379–388.

Cacciatore, J., Schnebly, S., & Froen, J. F. (2009). The effects of social support on maternal anxiety and depression after stillbirth. *Health & Social Care in the Community, 17*(2), 167–176.

Caldwell, B. A., & Redeker, N. S. (2009). Sleep patterns and psychological distress in women living in an inner city. *Research in Nursing & Health, 32*, 177–190.

Caleyachetty, R., Uthman, O. A., Bekele, H. N., Martin-Canavate, R., Marais, D., Coles, J., Steele, B., Uauy, R., & Koniz-Booher, P. (2019). Maternal exposure to intimate partner violence and breastfeeding practices in 51 low-income and middle-income countries: A population-based cross-sectional study. *PLoS Medicine, 16*(10), e1002921. https://doi.org/10.1371/journal.pmed.1002921

Cameron, E. E., Sedov, I. D., & Tomfohr-Madsen, L. (2016). Prevalence of paternal depression in pregnancy and the postpartum: An updated meta-analysis. *Journal of Affective Disorders, 206*, 189–203. https://doi.org/https://doi.org/10.1016/j.jad.2016.07.044

Canivet, C., Jakobsson, I., & Hagander, B. (2002). Colicky infants according to maternal reports in telephone interviews and diaries: A large Scandinavian study. *Journal of Developmental & Behavioral Pediatrics, 23*, 1–8.

Cappelletti, M., Della Bella, S., Ferrazzi, E., Mavilio, D., & Divanovic, S. (2016). Inflammation and preterm birth. *Journal of Leukocyte Biology, 99*, 67–78. https://doi.org/10.1189/jlb.3MR0615-272RR

Centers for Disease Control. (2019). *Infant mortality.* www.cdc.gov/reproductivehealth/maternalinfanthealth/infantmortality.htm

Centers for Disease Control and Prevention. (2015). *Mental health among women of reproductive age.* www.cdc.gov/reproductivehealth/depression/pdf/mental_health_women_repo_age.pdf

Cerulli, C., Talbot, N. L., Tang, W., & Chaudron, L. H. (2011). Co-occurring intimate partner violence and mental health diagnoses in perinatal women. *Journal of Women's Health, 20*, 1797–1803.

Chalise, A., & Bhandari, T. R. (2019). Postpartum depression and its associated factors: A community-based study in Nepal. *Journal of the Nepal Research Council, 17*(43), 200–205. https://doi.org/https://doi.org/10.33314/jnhrc.v0i0.1635

Chang, S.-R., Chen, K.-H., Ho, H.-N., Lai, Y.-H., Lin, M.-I., Lee, C.-N., & Lin, W.-A. (2015). Depressive symptoms, pain, and sexual dysfunction over the first year following vaginal or cesarean delivery. *International Journal of Nursing Studies, 52,* 1433–1444.

Chaudron, L. H., Klein, M. H., Remington, P., Palta, M., Allen, C., & Essex, M. J. (2001). Predictors, prodromes, and incidence of postpartum depression. *Journal of Psychosomatic Obstetrics & Gynecology, 22,* 103–112.

Chen, M., & Lacey, R. E. (2018). Adverse childhood experiences and adult inflammation: Findings from the 1958 British birth cohort. *Brain, Behavior & Immunity, 69,* 582–590. https://doi.org/10.1016/j.bbi.2018.02.007

Cheng, C.-Y., Chou, Y.-H., Chang, C.-H., & Liou, S.-R. (2021). Trends of perinatal stress, anxiety, and depression and their prediction on postpartum depression. *International Journal of Environmental Research and Public Health, 18,* 9307. https://doi.org/https://doi.org/10.3390/ijerph18179307

Choi, K. R., & Seng, J. S. (2016). Predisposing and precipitating factors for dissociation during labor in a cohort study of posttraumatic stress disorder and childbearing outcomes. *Journal of Midwifery and Women's Health, 61,* 68–76.

Chojenta, C. L., Lucke, J. C., Forder, P. M., & Loxton, D. (2016). Maternal health factors as risks for postnatal depression: A prospective longitudinal study. *PLoS One, 11*(1), e0147246. https://doi.org/10.1371/journal.pone.0147246

Christl, B., Reilly, N., Smith, M., Sims, D., Chavasse, F., & Austin, M.-P. (2013). The mental health of mothers of unsettled infants: Is there value in routine psychosocial assessment in this context? *Archives of Women's Mental Health, 16,* 391–399.

Clark, C. T., & Wisner, K. L. (2018). Treatment of peripartum bipolar disorder. *Obstetric & Gynecology Clinics of North America, 45,* 403–417. https://doi.org/https://doi.org/10.1016/j.ogc.2018.05.002

Collins, C. H., Zimmerman, C., & Howard, L. M. (2011). Refugee, asylum seeker, immigrants women and postnatal depression: Rates and risk factors. *Archives of Women's Mental Health, 14,* 3–11.

Coo, S., Garcia, M. I., Mira, A., & Valdes, V. (2020). The role of perinatal anxiety and depression in breastfeeding practices. *Breastfeeding Medicine, 15*(8), 495–500. https://doi.org/10.1089/bfm.2020.0091

Cook, N., Ayers, S., & Horsch, A. (2018). Maternal posttraumatic stress disorder during the perinatal period and child outcomes: A systematic review. *Journal of Affective Disorders, 225,* 18–35. https://doi.org/10.1016/j.jad.2017.07.045

Cooklin, A. R., Amir, L. H., Nguyen, C. D., Buck, M. L., Cullinane, M., Fisher, J. R. W., Donath, S. M., & CASTLE Study Team. (2018). Physical health, breastfeeding problems and maternal mood in the early postpartum: A prospective cohort study. *Archives of Women's Mental Health, 21*(3), 365–374. https://doi.org/10.1007/s00737-017-0805-y

Corwin, E. J., & Arbour, M. (2007). Postpartum fatigue and evidence-based interventions. *MCN, 32*(4), 215–220.

Corwin, E. J., Bozoky, I., Pugh, L. C., & Johnston, N. (2003). Interleukin-1 beta elevation during the postpartum period. *Annals of Behavioral Medicine, 25,* 41–47.

Corwin, E. J., Guo, Y., Pajer, K., Lowe, N., McCarthy, D., Schmiege, S., Weber, M., Pace, T., & Stafford, B. (2013). Immune dysregulation and glucocorticoid resistance in minority and low-income pregnant women. *Psychoneuroendocrinology, 38,* 1786–1796. https://doi.org/10.1016/j.psyneuen.2013.02.015

Corwin, E. J., & Johnston, N. (2008). Symptoms of postpartum depression associated with elevated levels of interleukin-1 beta during the first month postpartum. *Biological Research for Nursing, 10,* 128–133.

Corwin, E. J., & Pajer, K. (2008). The psychoneuroimmunology of postpartum depression. *Journal of Women's Health, 17*(9), 1529–1534.

Corwin, E. J., Pajer, K., Paul, S., Lowe, N., Weber, M., & McCarthy, D. O. (2015). Bidirectional psychoneuroimmune interactions in the early postpartum period influence risk of postpartum depression. *Brain, Behavior & Immunity*, *49*, 86–93. https://doi.org/10.1016/j.bbi2015.04.012

Coussons-Read, M. E., Lobel, M., Carey, J. C., Kreither, M. O., D'Anna, K., Argys, L., Ross, R. G., Brandt, C., & Cole, S. (2012). The occurrence of preterm delivery is linked to pregnancy-specific distress and elevated inflammatory markers across gestation. *Brain, Behavior & Immunity*, *26*, 650–659.

Coussons-Read, M. E., Okun, M. L., Schmitt, M. P., & Giese, S. (2005). Prenatal stress alters cytokine levels in a manner that may endanger human pregnancy. *Psychosomatic Medicine*, *67*, 625–631.

Creech, S. K., Kroll-Desrosiers, A. R., Benzer, J. K., Pulverman, C. S., & Mattocks, K. (2022). The impact of military sexual trauma on parent-infant bonding in a sample of perinatal women veterans. *Depression & Anxiety*, *39*(3), 201–210. https://doi.org/10.1002/da.23218

Crouch, J. L., Skowronski, J. J., Milner, J. S., & Harris, B. (2008). Parental responses to infant crying: The influence of child physical abuse risk and hostile priming. *Child Abuse & Neglect*, *32*, 702–710.

Da Costa, D., Dritsa, M., Verreault, N., Balaa, C., Kudzman, J., & Khalife, S. (2010). Sleep problems and depressed mood negatively impact health-related quality of life during pregnancy. *Archives of Women's Mental Health*, *13*, 249–257.

Dagher, R. K., McGovern, P. M., Alexander, B. H., Dowd, B. E., Ukestad, L. K., & McCaffrey, D. J. (2009). The psychosocial work environment and maternal postpartum depression. *International Journal of Behavioral Medicine*, *16*(4), 339–346. https://doi.org/10.1007/s12529-008-9014-4

Dagher, R. K., & Shenassa, E. D. (2012). Prenatal health behaviors and postpartum depression: Is there an association? *Archives of Women's Mental Health*, *15*, 31–37.

Danese, A., Moffitt, T. E., Harrington, H., Milne, B. J., Polanczyk, G., Pariante, C. M., & Caspi, A. (2009). Adverse childhood experiences and adult risk factors for age-related disease: Depression, inflammation, and clustering of metabolic risk factors. *Archives of Pediatric and Adolescent Medicine*, *163*(12), 1135–1143.

Danese, A., Pariante, C. M., Caspi, A., Taylor, A., & Poulton, R. (2007). Childhood maltreatment predicts adult inflammation in a life-course study. *Proceedings of the National Academy of Sciences USA*, *104*(4), 1319–1324. https://doi.org/0610362104 [pii] 10.1073/pnas.0610362104

Daoud, N., O'Brien, K., O'Campo, P., Harney, S., Harney, E., Bebee, K., Bourgeois, C., & Smylie, J. (2019). Postpartum depression prevalence and risk factors among Indigenous, non-Indigenous, and immigrant women in Canada. *Canadian Journal of Public Health*, *110*, 440–452. https://doi.org/https://doi.org/10.17269/s41997-019-00182-8

Daoud, N., Saleh-Darawshy, N. A., Gao, M., Sergienko, R., Sestito, S. R., & Geraisy, N. (2019). Multiple forms of discrimination and postpartum depression among indigenous Palestinian-Arab, Jewish immigrants and non-immigrant Jewish mothers. *BMC Public Health*, *19*, 1741. https://doi.org/https://doi.org/10.1186/s12889-019-8053-x

Darwin, Z., Domoney, J., Iles, J., Bristow, F., Siew, J., & Sethna, V. (2021). Assessing the mental health of fathers, other co-parents, and partners in the perinatal period: Mixed methods evidence synthesis. *Frontiers in Psychiatry*, *11*, 585479. https://doi.org/10.3389/fpsyt.2020.585479

Davidson, E. L., & Ollerton, R. L. (2020). Partners behaviours improving breastfeeding outcomes: An integrative review. *Women & Birth*, *33*(1), e15–e25. https://doi.org/10.1016/j.wombi.2019.05.010

Declercq, E. R., Sakala, C., Corry, M. P., & Applebaum, S. (2008). *New mothers speak out: National survey results highlight women's postpartum experiences*. Childbirth Connection.

de Jonge, P., Ormel, J., van den Brink, R. H., van Melle, J. P., Spijkerman, T. A., Kuijper, A., van Veldhuisen, D. J., van den Berg, M. P., Honig, A., Crijns, H. J., & Schene, A. H. (2006). Symptom dimensions of depression following myocardial infarction and their relationship with somatic health status and cardiovascular prognosis. *American Journal of Psychiatry*, *163*(1), 138–144. https://doi.org/163/1/138 [pii] 10.1176/appi.ajp.163.1.138

de Montigny, F., Girard, M. E., Lacharite, C., Dubeau, D., & Devault, A. (2013). Psychosocial factors associated with paternal postnatal depression. *Journal of Affective Disorders*, *150*(1), 44–49. https://doi.org/10.1016/j.jad.2013.01.048

Dennis, C.-L. (2004). Influence of depressive symptomatology on maternal health service utilization and general health. *Archives of Women's Mental Health*, *7*, 183–191.

Dennis, C.-L., Merry, L., Stewart, D., & Gagnon, A. J. (2016). Prevalence, continuation, and identification of postpartum depressive symptomatology among refugee, asylum-seeking, non-refugee immigrant, and Canadian-born women: Results from a prospective cohort study. *Archive of Women's Mental Health*, *19*, 959–967. https://doi.org/10.1007/s00737-016-0633-5

Dennis, C.-L., & Ross, L. E. (2005). Relationships among infant sleep patterns, maternal fatigue, and development of depressive symptomatology. *Birth*, *32*(3), 187–193.

Dennis, C.-L., & Ross, L. E. (2006a). The clinical utility of maternal self-reported personal and familial psychiatric history in identifying women at risk for postpartum depression. *Acta Obstetricia et Gynecologica*, *85*, 1179–1185.

Dennis, C.-L., & Ross, L. E. (2006b). Women's perceptions of partner support and conflict in the development of postpartum depressive symptoms. *Journal of Advanced Nursing*, *56*(6), 588–599.

de Schepper, S., Vercauteren, T., Tersago, J., Jacquemyn, Y., Raes, F., & Franck, E. (2016). Post-traumatic stress disorder after childbirth and the influence of maternity team care during labour and birth: A cohort study. *Midwifery*, *32*, 87–92.

des Rivieres-Pigeon, C., Seguin, L., Goulet, L., & Descarries, F. (2001). Unraveling the complexities of the relationship between employment status and postpartum depressive symptomatology. *Women & Health*, *34*, 61–79.

Dhabhar, F. D., & McEwen, B. S. (2001). Bidirectional effects of stress and glucocorticoid hormones on immune function: Possible explanations for paradoxical observations. In R. Ader, D. L. Felten, & N. Cohen (Eds.), *Psychoneuroimmunology* (3rd ed., Vol. 1, pp. 301–338). Academic Press.

Diamond, R. M., & Colainanni, A. (2022). The impact of perinatal healthcare changes on birth trauma during COVID-19. *Women & Birth*, *35*, 503–510. https://doi.org/https://doi.org/10.1016/j.wombi.2021.12.003

Dias, C. C., & Figueiredo, B. (2020). Mother's prenatal and postpartum depression symptoms in infant's sleep problems at 6 months. *Infant Mental Health Journal*, *41*, 614–627. https://doi.org/10.1002/imhj.21869

Di Blasio, P., Camisasca, E., & Maragoli, S. (2018). Childbirth related posttraumatic stress symptoms and maternal sleep difficulties: Associations with parenting stress. *Frontiers in Psychology*, *9*, 2103. https://doi.org/10.3389/fpsyg.2018.02103

Dikmen-Yildiz, P., Ayers, S., & Phillips, L. (2017). Factors associated with posttraumatic stress symptoms (PTSS) 4–6 weeks and 6 months after birth: A longitudinal population-based study. *Journal of Affective Disorders*, *221*, 238–245.

Ding, T., Wang, D. X., Chen, Q., & Zhu, S. N. (2014). Epidural labor analgesia is associated with a decreased risk of postpartum depression: A prospective cohort study. *Anesthesia & Analgesia*, *119*(2), 383–392. https://doi.org/10.1213/ANE.0000000000000107

Doan, T., Gardiner, A., Gay, C. L., & Lee, K. A. (2007). Breastfeeding increases sleep duration of new parents. *Journal of Perinatal & Neonatal Nursing*, *21*(3), 200–206.

Doke, P. P., Valdya, V. M., Narula, A. P. S., Datar, M. C., Patil, A. V., Panchanadikar, T. M., & Wagh, G. N. (2021). Assessment of difference in postpartum depression among caesarean and vaginally delivered women at 6-week follow-up in hospitals in Pune District, India: An observational cohort study. *BMJ Open*, *11*, e052008. https://doi.org/10.1136/bmjopen-2021-052008

Dol, J., Richardson, B., Grant, A., Aston, M., McMillan, D., Murphy, G. T., & Campbell-Yeo, M. (2021). Influence of parity and infant age on maternal self-efficacy, social support, postpartum anxiety, and postpartum depression in the first six months in the Maritime Provinces, Canada. *Birth*, *48*, 436–447. https://doi.org/10.1111/birt.12553

Dombrowski, M. A., Anderson, G. C., Santori, C., & Burkhammer, M. (2001). Kangaroo (skin-to-skin) care with a postpartum woman who is depressed. *MCN American Journal of Maternal-Child Nursing*, 26, 214–216.

Dorheim, S. K., Bondevik, G. T., Eberhard-Gran, M., & Bjorvatn, B. (2009a). Sleep and depression in postpartum women: A population-based study. *Sleep*, 32(7), 847–855.

Dorheim, S. K., Bondevik, G. T., Eberhard-Gran, M., & Bjorvatn, B. (2009b). Subjective and objective sleep among depressed and non-depressed postnatal women. *Acta Psychiatrica Scandinavia*, 119, 128–136.

Duan, Z., Wang, Y., Jiang, P., Wilson, A. E., Guo, Y., Lv, Y., Yang, X., Yu, R., Wang, S., Wu, Z., Xia, M., Wang, G., Tao, Y., Xiaohong, L., Ma, L., Shen, H., Sun, J., Deng, W., Yang, Y., & Chen, R. (2020). Postpartum depression in mothers and fathers: A structural equation model. *BMC Pregnancy and Childbirth*, 20, 537. https://doi.org/https://doi.org/10.1186/s12884-020-03228-9

Dubois, B. (2003). Overcoming the past. *New Beginnings*, March–April, 50–51.

Duivis, H. E., Kupper, N., Vermunt, J. K., Penninx, B. W., Bosch, N. M., Riese, H., Oldehinkel, A. J., & de Jonge, P. (2015). Depression trajectories, inflammation, and lifestyle factors in adolescence: The Tracking Adolescents' Individual Lives Survey. *Health Psychology*, 34(11), 1047–1057. https://doi.org/http://dx.doi.org/10.1037/hea0000210

Dunham, C. (1992). *Mamatoto: A celebration of birth*. Viking Penguin.

Eberhard-Gran, M., Garthus-Niegel, S., Garthus-Niegel, K., & Eskild, A. (2010). Postnatal care: A cross-cultural and historical perspective. *Archives of Women's Mental Health*, 13, 459–466.

Eisenach, J. C., Pan, P. H., Smiley, R., Lavand'homme, P., Landau, R., & Houle, T. T. (2008). Severity of acute pain after childbirth, but not type of delivery, predicts persistent pain and postpartum depression. *Pain*, 140, 87–94.

Elmir, R., Schmied, V., Wilkes, L., & Jackson, D. (2010). Women's perceptions and experiences of a traumatic birth: A meta-ethnography. *Journal of Advanced Nursing*, 66(10), 2142–2153.

Enlow, M. B., Kitts, R. L., Blood, E., Bizarro, A., Hofmeister, M., & Wright, R. J. (2011). Maternal posttraumatic stress symptoms and infant emotional reactivity and emotion regulation. *Infant Behavior & Development*, 34(4), 487–503.

Ertel, K. A., Koenen, K. C., Rich-Edwards, J. W., & Gillman, M. W. (2010). Antenatal and postpartum depressive symptoms are differentially associated with early childhood weight and adiposity. *Paediatric & Perinatal Epidemiology*, 24(2), 179–189.

Etain, B., Henry, C., Bellivier, F., Mathieu, F., & Leboyer, M. (2008). Beyond genetics: Childhood affective trauma in bipolar disorder. *Bipolar Disorders*, 10, 867–876.

Fagundes, C. P., Glaser, R., Hwang, B. S., Malarkey, W. B., & Kiecolt-Glaser, J. K. (2013). Depressive symptoms enhance stress-induced inflammatory responses. *Brain, Behavior & Immunity*, 31, 172–176. https://doi.org/10.1016/j.bbi.2012.05.006

Fairbrother, N., Collardeau, F., Albert, A. Y. K., Challacombe, F. L., Thordarson, D. S., Woody, S. R., & Janssen, P. A. (2021). High prevalence and incidence of obsessive-compulsive disorder among women across pregnancy and the postpartum. *Journal of Clinical Psychiatry*, 82(2), 61–68. https://doi.org/10.4088/JCP.20m13398

Falah-Hassani, K., Shiri, R., Vigod, S. N., & Dennis, C.-L. (2015). Prevalence of postpartum depression among immigrant women: A systematic review and meta-analysis. *Journal of Psychiatric Research*, 70, 67–82.

Fallon, V., Groves, R., Halford, J. C. G., Bennett, K. M., & Harrold, J. A. (2016). Postpartum anxiety and infant-feeding outcomes. *Journal of Human Lactation*, 32(4), 740–758. https://doi.org/10.1177/0890334416662241

Farr, S. L., Dietz, P. M., O'Hara, M. W., Burley, K., & Ko, J. Y. (2014). Postpartum anxiety and comorbid depression in a population-based sample of women. *Journal of Women's Health (Larchmont)*, 23(2), 120–128. https://doi.org/10.1089/jwh.2013.4438

Feeley, N., Zelkowitz, P., Cormier, C., Charbonneau, L., Lacroix, A., & Papgeorgiou, A. (2011). Posttraumatic stress among mother of very low birthweight infants 6 months after discharge from the neonatal intensive care unit. *Applied Nursing Research*, 24, 114–117.

Feldman, R., Granat, A., Pariente, C., Kanety, H., Kuint, J., & Gilboa-Schechtman, E. (2009). Maternal depression and anxiety across the postpartum year and infant social engagement, fear regulation, and stress reactivity. *Journal of the American Academy of Child and Adolescent Psychiatry, 48*(9), 919–927.

Felitti, V. J., Anda, R. F., Nordenberg, D., Williamson, D. F., Spitz, A. M., Edwards, V., Koss, M. P., & Marks, J. S. (1998). Relationship of childhood abuse and household dysfunction to many of the leading causes of death in adults. The Adverse Childhood Experiences (ACE) study. *American Journal of Preventive Medicine, 14*(4), 245–258. https://doi.org/S0749379798000178

Ferrucci, L., Cherubini, A., Bandinelli, S., Bartali, B., Corsi, A., Lauretani, F., Martin, A., Andres-Lacueva, C., Senin, U., & Guralnik, J. M. (2006). Relationship of plasma polyunsaturated fatty acids to circulating inflammatory markers. *Journal of Clinical Endocrinology & Metabolism, 91*, 439–446.

Field, T. (2010). Postpartum depression effects on early interactions, parenting, and safety practices: A review. *Infant Behavior & Development, 31*(1), 1–6. https://doi.org/10.1016/j.infbeh.2009.10.005

Field, T., Diego, M., & Hernandez-Reif, M. (2006). Prenatal depression effects on the fetus and newborn: A review. *Infant Behavior & Development, 29*, 445–455.

Field, T., Diego, M., Hernandez-Reif, M., Figueiredo, B., Schanberg, S., & Kuhn, C. (2007). Sleep disturbance in depressed pregnant women and their newborns. *Infant Behavior & Development, 30*, 127–133.

Figueiredo, B., & Costa, R. (2009). Mothers' stress, mood, and emotional involvement with the infant: 3 months before and 3 months after childbirth. *Archives of Women's Mental Health, 12*, 143–153.

Figueiredo, B., Dias, C. C., Brandao, S., Canario, C., & Nunes-Costa, R. (2013). Breastfeeding and postpartum depression: State of the art review. *Jornal de Pediatria, 89*(4), 332–338.

Figueiredo, B., Pinto, T. M., & Costa, R. (2021). Exclusive breastfeeding moderates the association between prenatal and postpartum depression. *Journal of Human Lactation.* https://doi.org/10.1177/0890334421991051

Forcada-Guex, M., Borghini, A., Pierrehumbert, B., Ansermet, F., & Muller-Nix, C. (2011). Prematurity, maternal posttraumatic stress and consequences on the mother-infant relationship. *Early Human Development, 87*, 21–26.

Ford, E., & Ayers, S. (2009). Stressful events and support during birth: The effect on anxiety, mood, and perceived control. *Journal of Anxiety Disorders, 23*, 260–268.

Ford, E., & Ayers, S. (2012). Support during birth interacts with prior trauma and birth intervention to predict postnatal post-traumatic stress symptoms. *Psychology & Health, 26*(12), 1553–1570.

Freeman, M. P., Smith, K. W., Freeman, S. A., McElroy, S. L., Kmetz, G. F., Wright, R., & Keck, P. E., Jr. (2002). The impact of reproductive events on the course of bipolar disorder in women. *Journal of Clinical Psychiatry, 63*, 284–287.

Freeman, M. P., Wright, R., Watchman, M., Wahl, R. A., Sisk, D. J., Fraleigh, L., & Weibrecht, J. M. (2005). Postpartum depression assessments at well-baby visits: Screening feasibility, prevalence, and risk factors. *Journal of Women's Health, 14*(10), 929–935.

Fukui, N., Motegi, T., Wantanabe, Y., Hashijiri, K., Tsuboya, R., Ogawa, M., Sugai, T., Egawa, J., Enomoto, T., & Someya, T. (2021). Exclusive breastfeeding is not associated with maternal-infant bonding in early postpartum, considering depression, anxiety, and parity. *Nutrients, 13*, 1184. https://doi.org/https://doi.org/10.3390/nu13041184

Furuta, M., Sandall, J., Cooper, D., & Bick, D. (2016). Predictors of birth-related posttraumatic stress symptoms: Secondary analysis of a cohort study. *Archives of Women's Mental Health, 19*, 987–999.

Gagnon, A. J., & Stewart, D. E. (2014). Resilience in international migrant women following violence associated with pregnancy. *Archives of Women's Mental Health, 17*, 303–310. https://doi.org/10.1007/s00737-013-0392-5

Galea, S., Vlahov, D., Resnick, H., Ahern, J., Susser, E., Gold, J., Bucuvalas, M., & Kilpatrick, D. (2003). Trends of probable post-traumatic stress disorder in New York City after the September 11 terrorist attacks. *American Journal of Epidemiology, 158*, 514–524.

Gannan, R., Sword, W., Thabane, L., Newbold, B., & Black, M. (2016). Predictors of postpartum depression among immigrant women in the year after childbirth. *Journal of Women's Health, 25*, 155–165.

Garthus-Niegel, S., Horsch, A., Ayers, S., Junge-Hoffmeister, J., Weidner, K., & Eberhard-Gran, M. (2018). The influence of postpartum PTSD on breastfeeding: A longitudinal population-based study. *Birth, 45*(2), 193–201. https://doi.org/10.1111/birt.12328

Garthus-Niegel, S., von Soest, T., Knoph, C., Simonsen, T. B., Torgersen, L., & Eberhard-Gran, M. (2014). The influence of women's preferences and actual mode of delivery on posttraumatic stress symptoms following childbirth: A population-based, longitudinal study. *BMC Pregnancy and Childbirth, 14*, 191. www.biocentral.com/1471-2393/14/191

Gausia, K., Fisher, C., Ali, M., & Oosthuizen, J. (2009). Antenatal depression and suicidal ideation among rural Bangladeshi women: A community-based study. *Archives of Women's Mental Health, 12*, 351–358.

Gheorghe, M., Varin, M., Wong, S. L., Baker, M., Grywacheski, V., & Orpana, H. (2021). Symptoms of postpartum anxiety and depression among women in Canada: Findings from a national cross-sectional survey. *Canadian Journal of Public Health, 112*, 244–252. https://doi.org/https://doi.org/10.17269/s41997-020-00420-4

Ghosh, J. K. C., Wilhelm, M. H., Dunkel-Schetter, C., Lombardi, C. A., & Ritz, B. R. (2010). Paternal support and preterm birth, and the moderation of effects of chronic stress. *Archives of Women's Mental Health, 13*, 327–338.

Giallo, R., Cooklin, A., & Nicholson, J. M. (2014). Risk factors associated with trajectories of mothers' depressive symptoms across the early parenting period. *Archives of Women's Mental Health, 17*, 115–125.

Giallo, R., Pilkington, P., Borschmann, R., Seymour, M., Dunning, M., & Brown, S. (2018). The prevalence and correlates of self-harm ideation trajectories in Australian women from pregnancy to 4-years postpartum. *Journal of Affective Disorders, 229*, 152–158.

Giardinelli, L., Innocenti, A., Benni, L., Stefanini, M. C., Lino, G., Lunardi, C., & Svelto, V. (2012). Depression and anxiety in the perinatal period: Prevalence and risk factors in an Italian sample. *Archives of Women's Mental Health, 15*, 21–30.

Gila-Diaz, A., Carrillo, G. H., de Pablo, A. L. L., Arribas, S. M., & Ramior-Cortijo, D. (2020). Association between maternal postpartum depression, stress, optimism, and breastfeeding pattern in the first six months. *International Journal of Environmental Research and Public Health, 17*, 7153. https://doi.org/10.3390/ijerph17197153

Gill, H., El-Halabi, S., Majeed, A., Gill, B., Lui, L. M. W., Mansur, R. B., Lipsitz, O., Rodrigues, N. B., Phan, L., Chen-Li, D., McIntyre, R. S., & Rosenblat, J. D. (2020). The association between adverse childhood experiences and inflammation in patients with major depressive disorder: A systematic review. *Journal of Affective Disorders, 272*, 1–7. https://doi.org/10.1016/j.jad.2020.03.145

Glynn, L. M., Schetter, C. D., Hobel, C. J., & Sandman, C. A. (2008). Pattern of perceived stress and anxiety in pregnancy predicts preterm birth. *Health Psychology, 27*(1), 43–51.

Gomez-Baya, D., Gomez-Gomez, I., Dominguez-Salas, S., Rodriguez-Dominguez, C., & Motrico, E. (2022). The influence of lifestyles to cope with stress over mental health in pregnant and postpartum women during the COVID-19 pandemic. *Current Psychology*, 1–20. https://doi.org/10.1007/s12144-022-03287-5

Goyal, D., Gay, C. L., & Lee, K. A. (2007). Patterns of sleep disruption and depressive symptoms in new mothers. *Journal of Perinatal & Neonatal Nursing, 21*(2), 123–129.

Goyal, D., Gay, C. L., & Lee, K. A. (2009). Fragmented maternal sleep is more strongly correlated with depressive symptoms than infant temperament at three months postpartum. *Archives of Women's Mental Health, 12*, 229–237.

Grajeda, R., & Perez-Escamilla, R. (2002). Stress during labor and delivery is associated with delayed onset of lactation among urban Guatemalan women. *Journal of Nutrition, 132*, 3055–3060.

Grant, K.-A., McMahon, C., Austin, M.-P., Reilly, N., Leader, L., & Ali, S. (2009). Maternal prenatal anxiety, postnatal caregiving and infants' cortisol responses to the still-face procedure. *Developmental Psychobiology, 51*, 625–637.

Grazioli, R., & Terry, D. J. (2000). The role of cognitive vulnerability and stress in the prediction of postpartum depression. *British Journal of Clinical Psychology, 39*, 329–347.

Gregory, E. F., Butz, A. M., Ghazarian, S. R., Gross, S. M., & Johnson, S. B. (2015). Are unmet breastfeeding expectations associated with maternal depressive symptoms? *Academic Pediatrics, 15*, 319–325.

Grekin, R., & O'Hara, M. W. (2014). Prevalence and risk factors of postpartum posttraumatic stress disorder: A meta-analysis. *Clinical Psychology Review, 34*, 389–401.

Grigoriadis, S., Graves, L., Peer, M., Mamisashvili, L., Tomlinson, G., Vigod, S. N., Dennis, C.-L., Steiner, M., Brown, C., Cheung, A., Dawson, H., Rector, N. A., Guenette, M., & Richter, M. (2018). Maternal anxiety during pregnancy and the association with adverse perinatal outcomes: Systematic review and meta-analysis. *Journal of Clinical Psychiatry, 79*(5), 17r12011. https://doi.org/10.4088/JCP.17r12011

Grisbrook, M.-A., & Letourneau, N. (2021). Improving maternal postpartum mental health screening guidelines. *Canadian Journal of Public Health, 112*, 240–243. https://doi.org/https://doi.org/10.17269/s41997-020-00373-8

Groer, M. W., Davis, M. W., & Hemphill, J. (2002). Postpartum stress: Current concepts and the possible protective role of breastfeeding. *Journal of Obstetric, Gynecologic, & Neonatal Nursing, 31*(4), 411–417. www.ncbi.nlm.nih.gov/entrez/query.fcgi?cmd=Retrieve&db=PubMed&dopt=Citation&list_uids=12146930

Groër, M. W., & Morgan, K. (2007). Immune, health and endocrine characteristics of depressed postpartum mothers. *Psychoneuroendocrinology, 32*(2), 133–139.

Gross, G. M., Kroll-Desrosiers, A. R., & Mattocks, K. (2020). A longitudinal investigation of military sexual trauma and perinatal depression. *Journal of Women's Health, 29*(1), 38–45. https://doi.org/10.1089/jwh.2018.7628

Grote, N. K., Bridge, J. A., Gavin, A. R., Melville, J. L., Iyengar, S., & Katon, W. (2010). A meta-analysis of depression during pregnancy and the risk of preterm birth, low birth weight, and intrauterine growth restriction. *Archives of General Psychiatry, 67*, 1012–1024.

Grote, N. K., Katon, W., Russo, J., Lohr, M. J., Curran, M., Galvin, E., & Carson, K. (2015). Collaborative care for perinatal depression in socioeconomically disadvantaged women: A randomized trial. *Depression & Anxiety, 32*, 821–834.

Gueron-Sela, N., Shahar, G., Volkovich, E., & Tikotzky, L. (2021). Prenatal matenal sleep and trajectories of postpartum depression and anxiety symptoms. *Journal of Sleep Research, 30*. https://doi.org/10.1002/imhj.21869

Haga, S. M., Ulleberg, P., Slinning, K., Kraft, P., Steen, T. B., & Staff, A. (2012). A longitudinal study of postpartum depressive symptoms: Multilevel growth curve analyses of emotion regulation strategies, breastfeeding self-efficacy, and social support. *Archives of Women's Mental Health, 15*, 175–184.

Hahn-Holbrook, J., Cornwell-Hinrichs, T., & Anaya, I. (2018). Economic and health predictors of national postpartum depression prevalence: A systematic review, meta-analysis, and meta-regression of 291 studies from 56 countries. *Frontiers in Psychiatry, 8*. https://doi.org/10.3389/fpsyt.2017.00248

Hahn-Holbrook, J., & Haselton, M. (2014). Is postpartum depression a disease of modern civilization? *Current Directions in Psychological Science, 23*(6), 395–400. https://doi.org/10.1177/0963721414547736

Hahn-Holbrook, J., Haselton, M. G., Schetter, C. D., & Glynn, L. M. (2013). Does breastfeeding offer protection against maternal depressive symptomatology? A prospective study from pregnancy to 2 years after birth. *Archives of Women's Mental Health, 16*, 411–422.

Hahn-Holbrook, J., Little, E. E., & Abbott, M. (2021). Mothers are more sensitive to infant cues after breastfeeding compared to bottle-feeding with human milk. *Hormones & Behavior, 136*. https://doi.org/https://doi.org/10.1016/j.yhbeh.2021.105047

Hairston, I. S., Solnik-Menilo, T., Deviri, D., & Handelzalts, J. E. (2016). Maternal depressed mood moderates the impact of infant sleep on mother-infant bonding. *Archives of Women's Mental Health, 19*, 1029–1039.

Hale, T. W. (2021). *Hales's medications and mothers' milk* (19th ed.). Springer Publishing.

Hamdan, A., & Tamim, H. (2011). Psychosocial risk and protective factors for postpartum depression in the United Arab Emirates. *Archives of Women's Mental Health, 14*, 125–133.

Hammen, C., & Brennan, P. (2002). Interpersonal dysfunction in depressed women: Impairments independent of depressive symptoms. *Journal of Affective Disorders, 72*, 145–156.

Handlin, L., Jonas, W., Pettersson, M., Ejdeback, M., Ransjo-Arvidson, A.-B., Nissen, A., & Uvnas-Moberg, K. (2009). Effects of sucking and skin-to-skin contact on maternal ACTH and cortisol levels during the second day postpartum: Influences of epidural analgesia and oxytocin in the perinatal period. *Breastfeeding Medicine, 4*(4), 207–220.

Harville, E. W., Xiong, X., & Buekens, P. (2010). Disasters and perinatal health: A systematic review. *Obstetrical & Gynecological Survey, 65*(11), 713–728.

Harville, E. W., Xiong, X., Pridjian, G., Elkind-Hirsch, K., & Buekens, P. (2009). Postpartum mental health after Hurricane Katrina: A cohort study. *BMC Pregnancy and Childbirth, 9*, 21.

Hay, D. F., Pawlby, S., Water, C. S., & Sharp, D. (2008). Antepartum and postpartum exposure to maternal depression: Different effects on different adolescent outcomes. *The Journal of Child Psychology and Psychiatry, 49*(10), 1079–1088.

Healey, C., Morriss, R., Henshaw, C., Wadoo, O., Sajjad, A., Scholefield, H., & Kinderman, P. (2013). Self-harm in postpartum depression and referrals to a perinatal mental health team: An audit study. *Archives of Women's Mental Health, 16*, 237–245.

Heck, J. L. (2021). Postpartum depression in American Indian/Alaska native women: A scoping review. *MCN American Journal of Maternal-Child Nursing, 46*(1), 1–13.

Heinrichs, M., Meinlschmidt, G., Neumann, I., Wagner, S., Kirschbaum, C., Ehlert, U., & Hellhammer, D. H. (2001). Effects of suckling on hypothalamic-pituitary-adrenal axis responses to psychosocial stress in postpartum lactating women. *Journal of Clinical Endocrinology & Metabolism, 86*, 4798–4804.

Helle, N., Barkmann, C., & Bartz-Seel, J. (2015). Very low birthweight as a risk factor for postpartum depression four to six weeks post birth in mothers and fathers: Cross-sectional results from a controlled multicentre cohort study. *Journal of Affective Disorders, 180*, 154–161.

Henriques, T., Leite de Moraes, C., Reichenheim, M. E., de Azevedo, G. L., Coutinho, E. S. F., & Figueira, I. L. D. (2015). Postpartum posttraumatic stress disorder in a fetal high-risk maternity hospital in the city of Rio de Janeiro, Brazil. *Cadernos de Saude Publica, 31*(12), 1–11. https://doi.org/http://dx.doi.org/10.1590/0102-311X00030215

Hibbeln, J. R. (2002). Seafood consumption, the DHA content of mothers' milk and prevalence rates of postpartum depression: A cross-national, ecological analysis. *Journal of Affective Disorders, 69*, 15–29.

Holland, M. L., Thevenent-Morrison, K., Mittal, M., Nelson, A., & Dozier, A. M. (2017). Breastfeeding and exposure to past, current, and neighborhood violence. *Maternal & Child Health Journal*. https://doi.org/10.1007/s10995-017-2357-1

Horsch, A., Lalor, J., & Downe, S. (2020). Moral and mental health challenges faced by maternity staff during COVID-19 pandemic. *Psychological Trauma, 12*(S1), S141–S142.

Horsely, K., Nguyen, T.-V., Ditto, B., & Da Costa, D. (2019). The association between pregnancy-specific anxiety and exclusive breastfeeding status early in the postpartum period. *Journal of Human Lactation, 35*(4), 729–736. https://doi.org/10.1177/0890334419838482

Hossain, S. J., Roy, B. R., Hossain, A. T., Mehrin, F., Tipu, S. M. M. U., Tofail, F., El Arifeen, S., Tran, T., Fisher, J., & Hamadani, J. (2020). Prevalence of maternal postpartum depression, health-seeking behavior, and out of pocket payment for physical illness and cost coping mechanism of the poor families of Bangladesh: A rural community-based study. *International Journal of Environmental Research and Public Health, 17*. https://doi.org/10.3390/ijerph17134727

Houston, K. A., Kaimal, A. J., Nakagawa, S., Gregorich, S. E., Yee, L. M., & Kuppermann, M. (2015). Mode of delivery and postpartum depression: The role of patient preference. *American Journal of Obstetrics and Gynecology, 212*(2), e1–e7.

Howard, L. M., Oram, S., Galley, H., Trevillion, K., & Feder, G. (2013). Domestic violence and perinatal mental disorders: A systematic review and meta-analysis. *PLoS Medicine, 10*(5). https://doi.org/10.1371/journal.pmed.1001452

Howell, K. H., Miller-Graff, L. E., Gilliam, H. C., & Carney, J. R. (2021). Factors related to parenting confidence among pregnant women experiencing intimate partner violence. *Psychological Trauma, 13*(3), 385–393. https://doi.org/http://dx.doi.org/10.1037/tra0000985

Hsiao, B.-S. J., & Sibeko, L. (2021). Breastfeeding is inversely associated with allostatic load in postpartum women: Cross-sectional data from nationally representative U.S. women. *Journal of Nutrition, 151*(12), 3801–3810. https://doi.org/10.1093/jn/nxab302

Huang, C.-M., Carter, P. A., & Guo, J.-L. (2004). A comparison of sleep and daytime sleepiness in depressed and non-depressed mothers during the early postpartum period. *Journal of Nursing Research, 12*(4), 287–295.

Hutchens, B. F., Kearney, J., & Kennedy, H. P. (2017). Survivors of child maltreatment and postpartum depression: An integrative review. *Journal of Midwifery and Women's Health, 62*(6), 706–722. https://doi.org/10.1111/jmwh.12680

Hutton, E. K., Hannah, M. E., Ross, S., Joseph, K. S., Ohlsson, A., Asztalos, E. V., & Willan, A. (2016). Maternal outcomes at 3 months after planned cesarean section versus planned vaginal birth for twin pregnancies in the twin birth study: A randomised controlled trial. *British Journal of Obstetrics & Gynaecology, 123*, 644. https://doi.org/20.2222/1471-0528.13597

Iido, M., Horiuchi, S., & Nagamori, K. (2014). A comparison of midwife-led care versus obstetrician-led care for low-risk women in Japan. *Women & Birth, 27*, 202–207.

Illiadis, S. I., Comasco, E., Sylven, S., Hellgren, C., Poromaa, I. S., & Skalkidou, A. (2015). Prenatal and postpartum evening salivary cortisol levels in association with peripartum depressive symptoms. *PLoS One*. https://doi.org/10.1371/journal.pone.0135471

Islam, M. J., Broidy, L., Baird, K., & Mazerolle, P. (2017). Intimate partner violence around the time of pregnancy and postpartum depression: The experience of women of Bangladesh. *PLoS One, 12*(5), e0176211. https://doi.org/https://doi.org/10.1371/journal.pone.0176211

Jahromi, M. K., Zare, A., Taghizadeganazdeh, M., & Koshkaki, A. R. (2014). A study of marital satisfaction among non-depressed and depressed mothers after childbirth in Jahrom, Iran, 2014. *Global Journal of Health Science, 26*(7), 140–146. https://doi.org/10.5539/gjhs.v7n3p140

Jankowski, M., Broderick, T. L., & Gutkowska, J. (2020). The role of oxytocin in cardiovascular protection. *Frontiers in Psychology, 11*. https://doi.org/10.3389/fpsyg.2020.02139

Jaremka, L. M., Lindgren, M. E., & Kiecolt-Glaser, J. K. (2013). Synergistic relationships among stress, depression, and troubled relationships: Insights from psychoneuroimmunology. *Depression & Anxiety, 30*(4). https://doi.org/10.1002/da.22078

JayaSalengia, B. H., Rajeswari, S., & Nalini, S. J. (2019). The relationship between maternal confidence, infant temperament, and postpartum depression. *Iranian Journal of Nursing, 24*, 437–443. https://doi.org/10.4103/ijnmr.IJNMR_208_18

Johansson, M., Benderix, Y., & Svensson, I. (2020). Mothers' and fathers' lived experiences of postpartum depression and parental stress after childbirth: A qualitative study. *International Journal of Qualitative Studies on Health and Well-Being, 15*(1), 1722564. https://doi.org/https://doi.org/10.1080/17482631.2020.1722564

Jones, I., & Craddock, N. (2001). Familiarity of the puerperal trigger in bipolar disorder: Results of a family study. *American Journal of Psychiatry, 158*, 913–917.

Jones, N. A., McFall, B. A., & Diego, M. A. (2004). Patterns of brain electrical activity in infants of depressed mothers who breastfeed and bottle feed: The mediating role of infant temperament. *Biological Psychology, 67*, 103–124.

Jotzo, M., & Poets, C. F. (2005). Helping parents cope with the trauma of premature birth: An evaluation of a trauma-preventive psychological intervention. *Pediatrics, 115*, 915–919.

Kalogerpoulos, C., Burdayron, R., Laganiere, C., Beliveau, M.-J., Dubois-Comtois, K., & Pennestri, M.-H. (2021). Investigating the link between sleep and postpartum depression in fathers utilizing subjective and objective sleep measures. *Sleep Medicine: X, 3*, 100036. https://doi.org/ https://doi.org/10.1016/j.sleepx.2021.100036

Kapulsky, L., Christos, P., Ilagan, J., & Kocsis, J. (2021). The effects of ibuprofen consumption on incidence of postpartum depression. *Clinical Neuropharmacology, 44*(4), 117–122. https://doi. org/10.1097/WNF.0000000000000448

Karlstrom, A., Engstrom-Olofsson, R., Norbergh, K. G., Sjoling, M., & Hidlingsson, I. (2007). Postoperative pain after cesarean birth affects breastfeeding and infant care. *Journal of Obstetric, Gynecologic and Neonatal Nursing, 36*(5), 430–440.

Kashaninia, Z., Sajedi, F., Rahgozar, M., & Noghabi, F. A. (2008). The effect of Kangaroo care on behavioral responses to pain of an intramuscular injection in neonates. *Journal of Specialized Pediatric Nursing, 13*(4), 275–280.

Kastello, J. C., Jacobsen, K. H., Gaffney, K. F., Kodadek, M. P., Bullock, L. C., & Sharps, P. W. (2016). Posttraumatic stress disorder among low-income women exposed to perinatal intimate partner violence. *Archives of Women's Mental Health, 19*, 521–528.

Kendall-Tackett, K. A. (2007). A new paradigm for depression in new mothers: The central role of inflammation and how breastfeeding and anti-inflammatory treatments protect maternal mental health. *International Breastfeeding Journal, 2*, 6. https://doi.org/doi:10.1186/1746-4358-2-6

Kendall-Tackett, K. A. (2010). Long-chain omega-3 fatty acids and women's mental health in the perinatal period. *Journal of Midwifery and Women's Health, 55*(6), 561–567.

Kendall-Tackett, K. A. (2014). Childbirth-related posttraumatic stress disorder symptoms and implications for breastfeeding. *Clinical Lactation, 5*(2), 51–55.

Kendall-Tackett, K.A. (2018). *Phantom of the Opera: A social history of the world's most popular musical*. Praeclarus Press.

Kendall-Tackett, K. A. (2022). *Breastfeeding doesn't need to suck: Caring for your baby and your mental health*. American Psychological Association.

Kendall-Tackett, K. A., & Beck, C. T. (2022). Secondary traumatic stress and moral injury in maternity care providers: A narrative and exploratory review. *Frontiers in Global Women's Health, 3*. https://doi.org/10.3389/fgwh.2022.835811

Kendall-Tackett, K. A., Cong, Z., & Hale, T. W. (2010). Mother-infant sleep locations and nighttime feeding behavior: U.S. data from the survey of mothers' sleep and fatigue. *Clinical Lactation, 1*(1), 27–30.

Kendall-Tackett, K. A., Cong, Z., & Hale, T. W. (2011). The effect of feeding method on sleep duration, maternal well-being, and postpartum depression. *Clinical Lactation, 2*(2), 22–26.

Kendall-Tackett, K. A., Cong, Z., & Hale, T. W. (2013). Depression, sleep quality, and maternal well-being in postpartum women with a history of sexual assault: A comparison of breastfeeding, mixed-feeding, and formula-feeding mothers *Breastfeeding Medicine, 8*(1), 16–22.

Kendall-Tackett, K. A., Cong, Z., & Hale, T. W. (2015). Birth interventions related to lower rates of exclusive breastfeeding and increased risk of postpartum depression in a large sample. *Clinical Lactation, 6*(3), 87–97.

Kendall-Tackett, K. A., Cong, Z., & Hale, T. W. (2018). The impact of feeding method and infant sleep location on mother/infant sleep, maternal depression, and mothers' well-being. *Clinical Lactation, 9*(3), 117–124. https://doi.org/http://dx.doi.org/10.1891/2158-0782.9.3.117

Kendall-Tackett, K. A., & Ruglass, L. M. (2017). *Women's mental health across the lifespan*. Routledge.

Kendall-Tackett, K. A., Walker, M., & Genna, C. W. (Eds.). (2018). *Tongue-tie: Expert roundtable*. Praeclarus Press.

Keogh, E., Hughes, S., Ellery, D., Daniel, C., & Holdcroft, A. (2006). Psychosocial influences on women's experience of planned elective cesarean section. *Psychosomatic Medicine*, 68(1), 167–174. https://doi.org/68/1/167 [pii] 10.1097/01.psy.0000197742.50988.9e

Kersting, A., Dorsch, M., Wesselman, U., Ludorff, K., Witthaut, J., Ohrmann, P., Hornig-Franz, I., Klockenbusch, W., Harms, E., & Arolt, V. (2004). Maternal posttraumatic stress response after the birth of a very low-birth-weight infant. *Journal of Psychosomatic Research*, 57, 473–476.

Kersting, A., Kroker, K., Steinhard, J., Hoernig-Franz, I., Wesselmann, U., Luedorff, K., & Ohrmann, P. (2009). Psychological impact on women after second and third trimester termination of pregnancy due to fetal anomalies versus women after preterm birth: A 14-month follow up study. *Archives of Women's Mental Health*, 12, 193–201.

Khadka, R., Hong, S. A., & Chang, Y.-S. (2020). Prevalence and determinants of poor sleep quality and depression among postpartum women: A community-based study in Ramechhap District, Nepal. *International Health*, 12, 125–131. https://doi.org/10.1093/inthealth/ihz032

Khajehei, M., Doherty, M., Tilley, P. J., & Sauer, K. (2015). Prevalence and risk factors of sexual dysfunction in postpartum Australian women. *Journal of Sexual Medicine*, 12, 1415–1426.

Khalifa, D. S., Glavin, K., Bjertness, E., & Lien, L. (2015). Postnatal depression among Sudanese women: Prevalence and validation of the Edinburgh postnatal depression scale at 3 months postpartum. *International Journal of Women's Health*, 7, 677–684.

Kharel, S., Binod, R., & Mandira, M. (2020). Evaluation of postpartum stress in breastfeeding and non-breastfeeding mothers of Kathmandu, Nepal. *World Family Medicine*, 18(7), 32–37. https://doi.org/10.5742MEWFM.2020.93832

Kiecolt-Glaser, J. K., Derry, H. M., & Fagundes, C. P. (2015). Inflammation: Depression fans the flames and feasts on the heat. *American Journal of Psychiatry*, 172(11), 1075–1091. https://doi.org/10.1176/appi.ajp.2015.15020152

Kiecolt-Glaser, J. K., Loving, T. J., Stowell, J. R., Malarky, W. B., Lemeshow, S., Dickinson, S. L., & Glaser, R. (2005). Hostile marital interactions, proinflammatory cytokine production, and wound healing. *Archives of General Psychiatry*, 62, 1377–1384.

Kiernan, K., & Pickett, K. E. (2006). Marital status disparities in maternal smoking during pregnancy, breast feeding and maternal depression. *Social Science & Medicine*, 63(2), 335–346.

Kim, D. R., Sockol, L. E., Sammel, M. D., Kelly, C., Moseley, M., & Epperson, C. N. (2013). Elevated risk of adverse obstetric outcomes in pregnant women with depression. *Archives of Women's Mental Health*, 16, 475–482.

Kim, J. J., Choi, S. S., & Ha, K. (2008). A closer look at depression in mothers who kill their children: Is it unipolar or bipolar depression? *Journal of Clinical Psychiatry*, 69(10), 1625–1631.

Kim, Y., Bird, A., Peterson, E., Underwood, L., Morton, S. M. B., & Grant, C. C. (2020). Maternal antenatal depression and early childhood sleep: Potential pathways through infant temperament. *Journal of Pediatric Psychology*, 45(2), 203–217. https://doi.org/10.1093/jpepsy/jsaa001

Kirpinar, I., Gozum, S., & Pasinlioglu, T. (2010). Prospective study of postpartum depression in eastern Turkey prevalence, socio-demographic and obstetric correlates, prenatal anxiety and early awareness. *Journal of Clinical Nursing*, 19, 422–431.

Kitzman-Ulrich, H., Wilson, D. K., Van Horn, M. L., & Lawman, H. G. (2010). Relationship of body mass index and psychosocial factors on physical activity in underserved adolescent boys and girls. *Health Psychology*, 29(5), 506–513.

Klainin, P., & Arthur, D. G. (2009). Postpartum depression in Asian cultures: A literature review. *International Journal of Nursing Studies*, 46, 1355–1373. https://doi.org/https://doi.org/10.1016/j.ijnurstu.2009.02.012

Knipscheer, J. W., & Kleber, R. J. (2006). The relative contribution of posttraumatic and acculturative stress to subjective mental health among Bosnian refugees. *Journal of Clinical Psychology*, 62, 339–353.

Kokubu, M., Okano, T., & Sugiyama, T. (2012). Postnatal depression, maternal bonding failure, and negative attitudes towards pregnancy: A longitudinal study of pregnant women in Japan. *Archive of Women's Mental Health, 15*, 221–216.

Koleva, H., & Stuart, S. (2014). Risk factors for depressive symptoms in adolescent pregnancy in a late-teen subsample. *Archives of Women's Mental Health, 17*, 155–159.

Kossakowska, K. (2018). Symptoms of postpartum depression and breastfeeding self-efficacy. *Pediatria Polska, 93*(2), 107–116. https://doi.org/ttps://doi.org/10.5114/polp.2018.76246

Koutra, K., Vassilaki, M., Georgiou, V., Koutis, A., Bitsios, P., Kogevinas, M., & Chatzi, L. (2018). Pregnancy, perinatal, and postpartum complications as determinants of postpartum depression: The Rhea mother-child cohort in Crete, Greece. *Epidemiology and Psychiatric Sciences, 27*(3), 244–255. https://doi.org/10.1017/S2045796016001062

Kritsotakis, G., Vassilaki, M., Melaki, V., Georgiou, V., Philalithis, A. E., Bitsios, P., & Kogevinas, M. (2013). Social capital in pregnancy and postpartum depressive symptoms: A prospective mother-child cohort study (the Rhea study). *International Journal of Nursing Studies, 50*, 63–72.

Krol, K. M., Rajhans, P., Missana, M., & Grossman, T. (2015). Duration of exclusive breastfeeding is associated with differences in infants' brain responses to emotional body expressions. *Frontiers in Behavioral Neuroscience, 8*, 459. https://doi.org/10.3389/fnbeh.2014.00459

Kroll-Desrosiers, A. R., Nephew, B. C., Babb, J. A., Guilarte-Walker, Y., Moore Simas, T. A., & Deligiannidis, K. M. (2017). Association of peripartum synthetic oxytocin administration and depressive anxiety disorders within the first postpartum year. *Depression & Anxiety, 34*(2), 137–142.

Kuo, S.-Y., Chen, S.-R., & Tzeng, Y.-L. (2014). Depression and anxiety trajectories among women who undergo an elective cesarean section. *PLoS One, 9*(1), e86653. https://doi.org/10.1371/journal.pone.0086653

Lane, R. D., Waldstein, S. R., Critchley, H. D., Derbyshire, S. W. G., Drossman, D. A., Wager, T. D., Schneiderman, N., Chesney, M. A., Jennings, J. R., Lovallo, W. R., Rose, R. M., Thayer, J. F., & Cameron, O. G. (2009). The rebirth of neuroscience in psychosomatic medicine, part II: Clinical applications and implications for research. *Psychosomatic Medicine, 71*, 135–151.

Lara-Cinisomo, S., McKenney, K., DiFlorio, A., & Meltzer-Brody, S. (2017). Associations between postpartum depression, breastfeeding, and oxytocin levels in Latina mothers. *Breastfeeding Medicine, 12*(7), 436–442. https://doi.org/10.1089/bfm.2016.0213

Lau, Y., & Chan, K. S. (2007). Influence of intimate partner violence during pregnancy and early postpartum depressive symptoms on breastfeeding among Chinese women in Hong Kong. *Journal of Midwifery and Women's Health, 52*(2), e15–e20.

Lauderdale, D. S. (2006). Birth outcomes for Arabic-named women in California before and after September 11. *Demography, 43*, 185–201.

Lee, S.-Y., Lee, K. A., Rankin, S. H., Weiss, S. J., & Alkon, A. (2007). Sleep disturbance, fatigue, and stress among Chinese-American parents with ICU hospitalized infants. *Issues in Mental Health Nursing, 28*, 593–605.

Leiferman, J. A., Farewell, C. V., Jewell, J., Lacy, R., Walls, J., Harnke, B., & Paulson, J. F. (2021). Anxiety among fathers during the prenatal and postpartum period: A meta-analysis. *Journal of Psychosomatic Obstetrics & Gynecology, 42*(2), 152–162. https://doi.org/10.1080/0167482X.2021.1885025

Letourneau, N., Duffett-Leger, L., Stewart, M., Hegadoren, K., Dennis, C.-L., Rinaldi, C. M., & Stoppard, J. (2007). Canadian mothers' perceived support needs during postpartum depression. *Journal of Obstetric, Gynecologic, and Neonatal Nursing, 36*, 441–449.

Letourneau, N. L., Dennis, C.-L., Benzies, K., Duffett-Leger, L., Stewart, M., Tryphonopoulos, P. D., Este, D., & Watson, W. (2012). Postpartum depression is a family affair: Addressing the impact on mothers, fathers, and children. *Issues in Mental Health Nursing, 33*, 445–457. https://doi.org/10.3109/01612840.2012.673054

Lev-Wiesel, R., Chen, R., Daphna-Tekoah, S., & Hod, M. (2009). Past traumatic events: Are they a risk factor for high-risk pregnancy, delivery complications, and postpartum posttraumatic symptoms? *Journal of Women's Health, 18*(1), 119–125.

Lewis, B. A., Gjerdingen, D. K., Schuver, K., Avery, M., & Marcus, B. H. (2018). The effect of sleep pattern changes on postpartum depressive symptoms. *BMC Women's Health*, 18, 12. https://doi.org/10.1186/s12905-017-0496-6

Li, Y., Long, Z., Cao, D., & Cao, F. (2017). Maternal history of child maltreatment and maternal depression risk in the perinatal period: A longitudinal study. *Child Abuse & Neglect*, 63, 192–201. https://doi.org/http://dx.doi.org/10.1016/j.chiabu.2016.12.001

Lim, G., LaSorda, K. R., Farrell, L. M., McCarthy, A. M., Facco, F., & Wasan, A. D. (2020). Obstetric pain correlates with postpartum depression symptoms: A pilot prospective observational study. *BMC Pregnancy and Childbirth*, 20(1), 240. https://doi.org/10.1186/s12884-020-02943-7

Liu, Y., Guo, N., Li, T., Zhuang, W., & Jiang, H. (2020). Prevalence and associated factors of postpartum anxiety and depression symptoms among women in Shanghai, China. *Journal of Affective Disorders*, 274, 848–856. https://doi.org/https://doi.org/10.1016/j.jad.2020.05.028

Logsdon, M. C., & Usui, W. (2001). Psychosocial predictors of postpartum depression in diverse groups of women. *Western Journal of Nursing Research*, 23, 563–574.

Lucas, A., Pizarro, E., Granada, M. L., Salinas, I., & Santmarti, A. (2001). Postpartum thyroid dysfunction and postpartum depression: Are they two linked disorders? *Clinical Endocrinology*, 55, 809–814.

Lui, Y., Zhang, L., Guo, N., & Jiang, H. (2021). Postpartum depression and postpartum post-traumatic stress disorder: Prevalence and associated factors. *BMC Psychiatry*, 21, 487. 10.1186/s12888-021-03432-7

Lupien, S. J., Parent, S., Evans, A. C., Tremblay, R. E., Zelazo, P., Corbo, V., Pruessner, J. C., & Seguin, J. R. (2011). Larger amygdala but no change in hippocampal volume in 10-year-old children exposed to maternal depressive symptomatology since birth. *Proceedings of the National Academy of Sciences USA*, 108(34), 14324–14329.

Machado, M. C., Assis, K. F., Oliveira, C., Ribeiro, A. Q., Araujo, R. M., Cury, A. F., Priore, S. E., & Franceschini, S. C. (2014). Determinants of the exclusive breastfeeding abandoment: Psychosocial factors. *Revista Saude Publica*, 48, 985–994.

Madeghe, B. A., Kimani, V. N., Vander Stoep, A., Nicodimos, S., & Kumar, M. (2016). Postpartum depression and infant feeding practices in a low income urban settlement in Nairobi-Kenya. *BMC Research Notes*, 9, 506. 10.1186/s13104-016-2307-9

Maehara, K., Mori, E., Sakajo, A., & Morita, A. (2017). Postpartum maternal function and parenting stress: Comparison by feeding methods. *International Journal of Nursing Practice*, 23(S1). https://doi.org/10.1111/ijn.12549

Maes, M. (2001). Psychological stress and the inflammatory response system. *Clinical Science*, 101, 193–194.

Maes, M., Lin, A., Ombelet, W., Stevens, K., Kenis, G., DeJongh, R., Cox, J., & Bosmans, E. (2000). Immune activation in the early puerperium is related to postpartum anxiety and depressive symptoms. *Psychoneuroendocrinology*, 25, 121–137.

Maes, M., Ombelet, W., DeJongh, R., Kenis, G., & Bosmans, E. (2001). The inflammatory response following delivery is amplified in women who previously suffered from major depression, suggesting that major depression is accompanied by a sensitization of the inflammatory response system. *Journal of Affective Disorders*, 63(1–3), 85–92.

Maes, M., & Smith, R. S. (1998). Fatty acids, cytokines, and major depression. *Biological Psychiatry*, 43, 313–314.

Mahenge, B., Stockl, H., Mizinduko, M., Mazalale, J., & Jahn, A. (2018). Adverse childhood experiences and intimate partner violence during pregnancy and their association to postpartum depression. *Journal of Affective Disorders*, 229, 159–163. https://doi.org/https://doi.org/10.1016/j.jad.2017.12.036

Maia, B. R., Pereira, A. T., Marques, M., Bos, S., Soares, M. J., Valente, J., & Gomes, A. A. (2012). The role of perfectionism in postpartum depression and symptomatology. *Archives of Women's Mental Health*, 15, 459–468.

Maina, G., Rosso, G., Aguglia, A., & Bogetto, F. (2014). Recurrence rates of bipolar disorder during the postpartum period: A study of 276 medication-free Italian women. *Archives of Women's Mental Health, 17*, 367–372.

Makrides, M., Gibson, R. A., & McPhee, A. J. (2010). Effect of DHA supplementation during pregnancy on maternal depression and neurodevelopment of young children: A randomized controlled trial. *Journal of the American Medical Association, 304*(15), 1675–1683.

Martinez-Torteya, C., Rosenblum, K. L., Katsonga-Phiri, T., Lindsay, H., & Muzik, M. (2018). Postpartum depression and resilience predict parenting sense of competence in women with childhood maltreatment history. *Archive of Women's Mental Health, 21*(6), 777–784. https://doi.org/10.1007/s00737-018-0865-7

Matijasevich, A., Murray, J., Cooper, P. J., Anselmi, L., Barros, A. J. D., Barros, F. C. F., & Santos, I. S. (2015). Trajectories of maternal depression and offspring psychopathology at 6 years: 2004 Pelotas cohort study. *Journal of Affective Disorders, 174*, 424–431.

Mauri, M., Oppo, A., Borri, C., & Banti, S. (2012). Suicidality in the perinatal period: Comparison of two self-report instruments. Results from PND-ReSeU. *Archives of Women's Mental Health, 15*, 39–47.

Mayopoulos, G. A., Ein-Dor, T., Dishy, G., Nandru, R., Chan, S. J., Hanley, L. E., Kaimal, A. J., & Dekel, S. (2021). COVID-19 is associated with traumatic childbirth and subsequent mother-infant bonding problems. *Journal of Affective Disorders, 282*, 122–125. https://doi.org/10.1016/j.jad.2020.12.101

Mazzeo, S. E., Slof-Op't Landt, M. C. T., Jones, I., Mitchell, K., Kendler, K. S., Neale, M. C., Aggen, S. H., & Bulik, C. M. (2006). Associations among postpartum depression, eating disorders, and perfectionism in a population-based sample of adult women. *International Journal of Eating Disorders, 39*(3), 202–211. https://doi.org/10.1002/eat

Mbah, A. K., Salihu, H. M., Dagne, G., Wilson, R. E., & Bruder, K. (2013). Exposure to environmental tobacco smoke and risk of antenatal depression. *Archives of Women's Mental Health, 16*, 293–302.

McCarter-Spaulding, D., & Horowitz, J. A. (2007). How does postpartum depression affect breastfeeding? *MCN, 32*(1), 10–17.

McCloskey, R. J. (2022). Postpartum physical health: The role of mothers' adverse childhood experiences and material hardship. *Psychological Trauma, 14*(8), 1272–1280. https://doi.org/https://doi.org/10.1037/tra0001137

McCoy, S. J., Beal, M., Shipman, S. B. M., Payton, M. E., & Watson, G. H. (2006). Risk factors for postpartum depression: A retrospective investigation at 4-weeks postnatal and a review of the literature. *Journal of the American Osteopathic Association, 106*, 193–198.

McGovern, P., Dowd, B. E., Gjerdingen, D., Gross, C. R., Kenney, S., Ukestad, L., McCaffrey, D., & Lundberg, U. (2006). Postpartum health of employed mothers 5 weeks after childbirth. *Annals of Family Medicine, 4*(2), 159–167.

McGrath, J. M., Records, K., & Rice, M. (2008). Maternal depression and infant temperament characteristics. *Infant Behavior & Development, 31*, 71–80.

McLearn, K. T., Minkovitz, C. S., Strobion, D. M., Marks, E., & Hou, W. (2006). Maternal depressive symptoms at 2 to 4 months postpartum and early parenting practices. *Archives of Pediatrics and Adolescent Medicine, 160*(3), 279–284.

Mehdi, S. F., Pusapati, S., Khenhrani, R. R., Farooqi, M. S., Sarwar, S., Alnasarat, A., Mathur, N., Metz, C. N., LeRoith, D., Tracey, K. J., Yang, H., Brownstein, M. J., & Roth, J. (2022). Oxytocin and related peptide hormones: Candidate anti-inflammatory therapy in early stages. *Frontiers in Immunology, 13*. 10.3389/fimmu.2022.864007.

Melrose, S. (2010). Paternal postpartum depression: How can nurses begin to help? *Contemporary Nurse, 34*(2), 199–210. https://doi.org/https://doi.org/10.5172/conu.2010.34.2.199

Mezzacappa, E. S., & Endicott, J. (2007). Parity mediates the association between infant feeding method and maternal depressive symptoms in the postpartum. *Archives of Women's Mental Health, 10*, 259–266.

Mezzavilla, R. D. S., Ferreira, M. D. F., Curloni, C. C., Lindsay, A. C., & Hasselman, M. H. (2018). Intimate partner violence and breastfeeding practices: A systematic review of observational studies. *Jornal de Pediatria*, 94, 226–237. https://doi.org/https://doi.org/10.1016/j.jped.2017.07.007

Mezzavilla, R. D. S., Vianna, G. V. D. B., Lindsay, A. C., & Hasselmann, M. H. (2021). Intimate partner violence, breastfeeding, breastmilk substitutes, and baby bottle use in the first year of life. *Ciencia & Saude Coletiva*, 26(5), 1955–1964. https://doi.org/10.1590/1413-81232021265.10012019

Middleton, P., Gomersall, J. C., Gould, J. F., Shepherd, E., Olsen, S. F., & Makrides, M. (2018, November 15). Omega-3 fatty acid addition during pregnancy. *Cochrane Database of Systematic Reviews*, 11(11), CD003402.

Miksic, S., Uglesic, B., Jakab, J., Holik, D., Srb, A. M., & Degmecic, D. (2020). Positive effect of breastfeeding on child development, anxiety, and postpartum depression. *International Journal of Environmental Research and Public Health*, 17, 2725. https://doi.org/10.3390/ijerph17082725

Miller, D. A., McClusky-Fawcett, K., & Irving, L. M. (1993). The relationship between childhood sexual abuse and subsequent onset of bulimia nervosa. *Child Abuse & Neglect*, 17, 305–314.

Miller, J. (2019). *Evidence-based chiropractic care for infants: Rationale, therapies, and outcomes.* Praeclarus Press.

Miller, J. (2020). Breastfeeding support team: When to add a chiropractor. *Clinical Lactation*, 11(1), 7–20.

Miszkurka, M., Zuzunegui, M. V., & Goulet, L. (2012). Immigrant status, antenatal depressive symptoms, and frequency and source of violence: What's the relationship. *Archives of Women's Mental Health*, 15, 387–396.

Mitchell, A. M., Porter, K., & Christian, L. M. (2018). Examination of the role of obesity in the association between childhood trauma and inflammation during pregnancy. *Health Psychology*, 37(2), 114–124. https://doi.org/https://doi.org/10.1037/hea0000559

Modarres, M., Afrasiabi, S., Rahnama, P., & Montazeri, A. (2012). Prevalence and risk factors of childbirth-related post-traumatic stress symptoms. *BMC Pregnancy and Childbirth*, 12, 88. www.biomedcentral.com/1471-2393/12/88

Molgora, S., Fenaroli, V., Malgaroli, M., & Saita, E. (2017). Trajectories of postpartum depression in Italian first-time fathers. *American Journal of Men's Health*, 11(4), 880–887. https://doi.org/10.1177/1557988316676692

Monti, F., Agostini, F., Fagandini, P., La Sala, G. B., & Blickstein, I. (2009). Depressive symptoms during late pregnancy and early parenthood following assisted reproductive technology. *Fertility & Sterility*, 91(3), 851–857.

Mora, P. A., Bennett, I. M., Elo, I. T., Mathew, L., Coyne, J. C., & Culhane, J. F. (2009). Distinct trajectories of perinatal depressive symptomatology: Evidence from growth mixing modeling. *American Journal of Epidemiology*, 169(1), 24–32.

Morgan, J. F., Lacey, J. H., & Chung, E. (2006). Risk of postnatal depression, miscarriage, and preterm birth in bulimia nervosa: Retrospective controlled study. *Psychosomatic Medicine*, 68, 487–492.

Moses-Kolko, E. L., Berga, S. L., Kalro, B., Sit, D. K. Y., & Wisner, K. L. (2009). Transdermal estradiol for postpartum: A promising treatment option. *Clinical Obstetrics & Gynecology*, 52, 516–529.

Moses-Kolko, E. L., & Roth, E. K. (2004). Antepartum and postpartum depression: Healthy mom, healthy baby. *Journal of the American Medical Women's Association*, 59, 181–191.

Munk-Olsen, T., Laursen, T. M., Mendelson, T., & Pedersen, C. B. (2010). Perinatal mental disorders in native Danes and immigrant women. *Archives of Women's Mental Health*, 13, 319–326.

Murray, L., Dunne, M. P., Vo, T. V., Anh, P. N. T., Khawaja, N. G., & Cao, T. N. (2015). Postnatal depressive symptoms amongst women in central Vietnam: A cross-sectional study investigating prevalence and associations with social, cultural, and infant factors. *BMC Pregnancy and Childbirth*, 15, 234.

Muzik, M., Bocknek, E. L., Broderick, A., Richardson, P., Rosenblum, K. L., Thelen, K., & Seng, J. S. (2013). Mother-infant bonding impairment across the first 6 months postpartum: The primacy of psychopathology in women with childhood abuse and neglect histories. *Archives of Women's Mental Health*, 16, 29–38.

Navarrete, L., Nieto, L., & Lara, M. A. (2021). Intimate partner violence and perinatal depression and anxiety: Social support as moderator among Mexican women. *Sexual & Reproductive Healthcare*, 27, 100569. https://doi.org/https://doi.org/10.1016/j.srhc.2020.100569

Navarro, P., Garcia-Esteve, L., Ascaso, C., Aguado, J., Gelabert, E., & Martin-Santos, R. (2008). Non-psychotic psychiatric disorders after childbirth: Prevalence and comorbidity in a community sample. *Journal of Affective Disorders*, 109, 171–176.

Netsi, E., Van Ijzendoorn, M., Bakermans-Kranenburg, M. J., Wulff, K., Jansen, P. W., Jaddoe, V. W., Verhulst, F. C., Tiemeier, H., & Ramchandani, P. G. (2015). Does infant reactivity moderate the association between antenatal maternal depression and infant sleep? *Journal of Developmental & Behavioral Pediatrics*, 36(6), 440–449.

Newland, R. P., Parade, S. H., Dickstein, S., & Seifer, R. (2016). Goodness of fit between prenatal maternal sleep and infant sleep: Associations with maternal depression and attachment security. *Infant Behavior & Development*, 44, 179–188.

Ngai, F.-W., & Ngu, S.-F. (2015). Predictors of maternal and paternal depressive symptoms at postpartum. *Journal of Psychosomatic Research*, 78, 156–161.

Nicklas, J. M., Miller, L. J., Zera, C. A., Davis, R. B., Levkoff, S. E., & Seely, E. W. (2013). Factors associated with depressive symptoms in the early postpartum period among women with recent gestational diabetes mellitus. *Maternal & Child Health Journal*, 17, 1665–1672. https://doi.org/10.1007/s10995-012-1180-y

Nillni, Y. I., Shayani, D. R., Finley, E., Copeland, L. A., Perkins, D. F., & Vogt, D. S. (2020). The impact of posttraumatic stress disorder and moral injury on women veterans' perinatal outcomes following separation from military service. *Journal of Traumatic Stress*, 33, 248–256. https://doi.org/10.1002/jts.22509

Nishigori, H., Obara, T., Nishigori, T., Metoki, H., Mizuno, S., Ishikuro, M., Sakurai, K., Hamada, H., Wantanabe, Z., & Miyagi Regional Center of Japan Environment and Children's Study Group. (2020). The prevalence and risk factors for postpartum depression symptoms of fathers at one and 6 months postpartum: An adjunct study of the Japan Environment & Children's Study. *Journal of Maternal-Fetal & Neonatal Medicine*, 33(16), 2797–2804. https://doi.org/https://doi.org/10.1080/14767058.2018.1560415

Nishimura, A., Fujita, Y., Katsuta, M., Ishihara, A., & Ohashi, K. (2015). Paternal postnatal depression in Japan: An investigation of correlated factors including relationship with partner. *BMC Pregnancy and Childbirth*, 15, 128. https://doi.org/10.1186/s12884-015-0552-x

Normann, A. K., Bakiewicz, A., Madsen, F. K., Khan, K. S., Rasch, V., & Linde, D. S. (2020). Intimate partner violence and breastfeeding: A systematic review. *BMJ Open*, 10(10), e034153. https://doi.org/10.1136/bmjopen-2019-034153

Nutor, J. J., Slaughter-Acey, J. C., Giurgescu, C., & Misra, D. P. (2018). Symptoms of depression and preterm birth among black women. *MCN American Journal of Maternal-Child Nursing*, 43(5), 252–258. https://doi.org/10.1097/NMC.0000000000000464

O'Donovan, A., Alcorn, K. L., Patrick, J. C., Creedy, D., Dawe, S., & Devilly, G. J. (2014). Predicting posttraumatic stress disorder after childbirth. *Midwifery*, 30, 935–941.

O'Higgins, M., James Roberts, I., St., Glover, M., & Taylor, A. (2013). Mother-child bonding at 1 year: Associations with symptoms of postnatal depression and bonding in the first few weeks. *Archives of Women's Mental Health*, 16, 381–389.

Okun, M. L., Mancuso, R. A., Hobel, C. J., Schetter, C. D., & Coussons-Read, M. E. (2018). Poor sleep quality increases symptoms of depression and anxiety in postpartum women. *Journal of Behavioral Medicine*, 41, 703–710. https://doi.org/https://doi.org/10.1007/s10865-018-9950-7

O'Leary, J. (2005). The trauma of ultrasound during a pregnancy following perinatal loss. *Journal of Loss and Trauma*, 10, 183–204.

Onoye, J. M., Goebert, D., Morland, L., & Matsu, C. (2009). PTSD and postpartum mental health in a sample of Caucasian, Asian, and Pacific Islander women. *Archives of Women's Mental Health, 12*, 393–400.

Onoye, J. M., Shafer, L. A., Goebert, D., Morland, L., Matsu, C., & Hamagami, F. (2013). Changes in PTSD symptomatology and mental health during pregnancy and postpartum. *Archives of Women's Mental Health, 16*, 453–463.

Orr, S. T., Reiter, J. P., Blazer, D. G., & James, S. A. (2007). Maternal prenatal pregnancy-related anxiety and spontaneous preterm birth in Baltimore, Maryland. *Psychosomatic Medicine, 69*, 566–570.

Osborne, L. M. (2018). Recognizing and managing postpartum psychosis. *Obstetric & Gynecology Clinics, 45*(3), 455–468.

Osborne, L. M., Voegline, K., Standeven, L. R., Sundel, B., Pangtey, M., Hantsoo, L., & Payne, J. L. (2021). High worry in pregnancy predicts postpartum depression. *Journal of Affective Disorders, 294*, 701–706. https://doi.org/https://doi.org/10.1016/j.jad.2021.07.009

Oyentunji, A., & Chandra, P. (2020). Postpartum stress and infant outcome: A review of current literature. *Psychiatry Research, 284*. https://doi.org/https://doi.org/10.1016/j.psychres.2020.112769

Pao, C., Guintivano, J., Santos, H., & Meltzer-Brody, S. (2019). Postpartum depression and social support in a racially and ethnically diverse population of women. *Archives of Women's Mental Health, 22*(1), 105–114. https://doi.org/10.1007/s00737-018-0882-6

Park, J.-H., Karmaus, W., & Zhang, H. (2015). Prevalence of and risk factors for depressive symptoms in Korean women throughout pregnancy and the postpartum period. *Asian Nursing Research, 9*, 219–225.

Parmar, V. R., Kumar, A., Kaur, R., Parmar, S., Kaur, D., Basu, S., Jain, S., & Narula, S. (2009). Experience with kangaroo mother care in a Neonatal Intensive Care Unit (NICU) in Chandigarh, India. *Indian Journal of Pediatrics, 76*(1), 25–28.

Paxson, C., Fussell, E., Rhodes, J., & Waters, M. (2010). Five years later: Recovery from post-traumatic stress and psychological distress among low-income mothers affected by Hurricane Katrina. *Social Science & Medicine, 74*, 150–157.

Pearson, R. M., Lightman, S. L., & Evans, J. (2012). Symptoms of depression during pregnancy are associated with increased systolic blood pressure responses towards infant distress. *Archives of Women's Mental Health, 15*, 95–105.

Pedersen, C. A., Johnson, J. L., Silva, S., Bunevicius, R., Meltzer-Brody, S., Hamer, M., & Leserman, J. (2007). Antenatal thyroid correlates of postpartum depression. *Psychoneuroendocrinology, 32*(3), 235–245.

Pedersen, S. C., Maindal, H. T., & Ryom, K. (2021, May-June). "I wanted to be there as a father, but I couldn't": A qualitative study of fathers' experiences of postpartum depression and their help-seeking behavior. *American Journal of Men's Health*, 1–13. https://doi.org/10.1177/15579883211024375

Pelaez, M., Field, T., Pickens, J. N., & Hart, S. (2008). Disengaged and authoritarian parenting behavior of depressed mothers with their toddlers. *Infant Behavior & Development, 31*, 145–148.

Plaza, A., Garcia-Esteve, L., Ascaso, C., Navarro, P., Gelabert, E., Halperin, I., Valdes, M., & Martin-Santos, R. (2010). Childhood sexual abuse and hypothalamus-pituitary-thyroid axis in postpartum major depression. *Journal of Affective Disorders, 122*, 159–163.

Pope, C. J., Xie, B., Sharma, V., & Campbell, M. K. (2013). A prospective study of thoughts of self-harm and suicidal ideation during the postpartum period in women with mood disorders. *Archives of Women's Mental Health, 16*, 483–388.

Porcel, J., Feigal, C., Poye, L., Postmas, I. R., Zeeman, G. G., Olowoyeye, A., Tsigas, E., & Wilson, M. (2013). Hypertensive disorders of pregnancy and risk of screening positive for posttraumatic stress disorder: A cross-sectional study. *Pregnancy Hypertension, 3*, 254–260.

Posmontier, B. (2008). Sleep quality in women with and without postpartum depression. *Journal of Obstetric, Gynecologic and Neonatal Nursing, 37*(6), 722–737.

H. Priddis, V. Schmied and H. Dahlen (2014). Women's experiences following severe perinatal trauma: A qualitative study. *BMC Women's Health*. *14*(32). www.biomedcentral.com/1472-6874/14/32

Prochaska, E. (2015). Human rights in maternity care. *Midwifery*, *31*, 1015–1016.

Punamaki, R. L., Diab, S. Y., Isosavi, S., Kuittinen, S., & Qouta, S. R. (2018). Maternal pre- and postnatal mental health and infant development in war conditions: The Gaza infant study. *Psychological Trauma*, *10*(2), 144–153. https://doi.org/http://dx.doi.org/10.1037/tra0000275

Putnick, D. L., Bell, E. M., Ghassabian, A., Mendola, P., Sundaram, R., & Yeung, E. H. (2022). Maternal antenatal depression's effects on child developmental delays: Gestational age, postnatal depressive symptoms, and breastfeeding as mediators. *Journal of Affective Disorders*. https://doi.org/https://doi.org/10.1016/j.jad.2022.12.059

Qu, Z., Wang, X., Tian, D., Zhao, Y., Zhang, Q., He, H., & Zhang, X. (2012). Posttraumatic stress disorder and depression among new mothers at 8 months after the 2008 Sichuan earthquake in China. *Archive of Women's Mental Health*, *15*, 49–55.

Rados, S. N., Tadinac, M., & Herman, R. (2018). Anxiety during pregnancy and postpartum course: Predictors and comorbidity with postpartum depression. *Acta Clinica Croatia*, *57*, 39–51. https://doi.org/10.20471/acc.2018.57.01.05

Ramakrishna, S., Cooklin, A. R., & Leach, L. S. (2019). Comorbid anxiety and depression: A community-based study examining symptomology and correlates during the postpartum period. *Journal of Reproductive and Infant Psychology*, *37*, 468–479. https://doi.org/https://doi.org/10.1080/02646838.2019.1578870

Rao, W.-W., Zhu, X.-M., Zong, Q.-Q., Zhang, Q., Hall, B. J., Ungvari, G. S., & Xiang, Y.-T. (2020). Prevalence of prenatal and postpartum depression in fathers: A comprehensive meta-analysis of observational studies. *Journal of Affective Disorders*, *263*, 491–499. https://doi.org/https://doi.org/10.1016/j.jad.2019.10.030

Reading, R., & Reynolds, S. (2001). Debt, social disadvantage and maternal depression. *Social Science & Medicine*, *53*, 441–453.

Reid, K. M., & Taylor, M. G. (2015). Social support, stress, and maternal postpartum depression: A comparison of supportive relationships. *Social Science & Medicine*, *54*, 246–262.

Rich-Edwards, J. W., James-Todd, T., Mohllajee, A., Kleinman, K., Burke, A., Gillman, M. W., & Wright, R. J. (2011). Lifetime maternal experiences of abuse and risk of pre-natal depression in two demographically distinct populations in Boston. *International Journal of Epidemiology*, *40*(2), 375–384.

Roberts, E., Norman, P., & Barton, J. (2016). Posttraumatic stress disorder following childbirth: A meta-ethnography. *Journal of Ethnographic & Qualitative Research*, *11*, 154–170.

Rodriguez, M. A., Valentine, J. M., Ahmed, S. R., Eisenman, D. P., Sumner, L. A., Heilemann, M. S., & Liu, H. (2010). Intimate partner violence and maternal depression during the perinatal period: A longitudinal investigation of Latinas. *Violence Against Women*, *16*(5), 543–559. https://doi.org/10.1177/1077801210366959

Rosenblum, K. L., McDonough, S., Muzik, M., Miller, A., & Sameroff, A. (2002). Maternal representations of the infant: Associations with infant response to the still face. *Child Development*, *73*, 999–1015.

Ross, L. E., & Dennis, C.-L. (2009). The prevalence of postpartum depression among women with substance use, an abuse history, or chronic illness: A systematic review. *Journal of Women's Health*, *18*(4), 475–486.

Ross, L. E., & McLean, L. M. (2006). Anxiety disorders during pregnancy and the postpartum period: A systematic review. *Journal of Clinical Psychiatry*, *67*, 1285–1298.

Ross, L. E., Murray, B. J., & Steiner, M. (2005). Sleep and perinatal mood disorders: A critical review. *Journal of Psychiatry & Neuroscience*, *30*, 247–256.

Rosseland, L. A., Reme, S. E., Simonsen, T. B., Thoresen, M., Nielsen, C. V., & Gran, M. E. (2020). Are labor pain and birth experience associated with persistent pain and postpartum depression? A prospective cohort study. *Scandinavian Journal of Pain, 20*(3), 591–602. https://doi.org/10.1515/sjpain-2020-0025

Roux, G., Anderson, C., & Roan, C. (2002). Postpartum depression, marital dysfunction, and infant outcome: A longitudinal study. *Journal of Perinatal Education, 11*, 25–36.

Rowlands, I. J., & Redshaw, M. (2012). Mode of birth and women's psychological and physical wellbeing in the postnatal period. *BMC Pregnancy and Childbirth, 12*, 138. www.biomedcentral.com/1471-2393/12/138

Runsten, S. (2013). Can social support alleviate inflammation associated with childhood adversities? *Nordic Journal of Psychiatry, 68*(2), 137–144. https://doi.org/10.3109/08039488.2013.786133

Sachs-Ericsson, N., Cromer, K., Hernandez, A., & Kendall-Tackett, K. A. (2009). Childhood abuse, health and pain-related problems: The role of psychiatric disorders and current life stress. *Journal of Trauma & Dissociation, 10*, 170–188.

Sampson, M., Yu, M., Mauldin, R., Mayorga, A., & Gonzales, L. G. (2021). "You withhold what you are feeling so you can have a family": Latinas' perceptions on community values and postpartum depression. *BMJ: Family Medicine & Community Health, 0*, e000504.

Sargent, C. (2015). *Birth trauma in New Zealand: Some major concerns*. Voice for Parents.

Sawada, N., Gagne, F. M., Seguin, L., Kramer, M. S., McNamara, H., Platt, R. W., Goulet, L., Meaney, M. J., & Lynch, J. E. (2015). Maternal prenatal felt security and infant health at birth interact to predict infant fussing and crying at 12 months postpartum. *Health Psychology, 34*(8), 811–819. https://doi.org/http://dx.doi.org/10.1037/hea0000152

Saxbe, D. E., Schetter, C. D., Guardino, C. M., Ramey, S. L., Shalowitz, M. U., Thorp, J., Vance, M., Shriver, E. K., & National Institute of Child Human Development Community Child Health Network. (2016). Sleep quality predicts persistence of parental postpartum depressive symptoms and transmission of depressive symptoms from mothers to fathers. *Annals of Behavioral Medicine, 50*(6), 862–875. https://doi.org/10.1007/s12160-016-9815-7

Schiller, C. E., O'Hara, M. W., Rubinow, D. R., & Johnson, A. K. (2013). Estradiol modulates anhedonia and behavioral despair in rats and negative affect in a subgroup of women at high risk for postpartum depression. *Physiology & Behavior, 119*, 137–144.

Schwartz, E. B., Ray, R. M., Stuebe, A. M., Allison, M. A., Ness, R. B., Freiberg, M. S., & Cauley, J. A. (2009). Duration of lactation and risk factors for maternal cardiovascular disease. *Obstetrics & Gynecology, 113*(5), 974–982.

Scorza, P., Owusu-Agyei, S., Asampong, E., & Wainberg, M. L. (2015). The expression of perinatal depression in rural Ghana. *International Journal of Cultural Mental Health, 8*, 370–381.

Seng, J. S. (2011). Disparity in posttraumatic stress disorder diagnosis among African American pregnant women. *Archives of Women's Mental Health, 14*(4), 295–306.

Seng, J. S., Low, L. K., Sperlich, M. A., Ronis, D. L., & Liberzon, I. (2011). Posttraumatic stress disorder, child abuse history, birth weight, and gestational age: A prospective cohort study. *British Journal of Obstetrics & Gynecology, 118*(11), 1329–1339.

Seng, J. S., Low, L. M. K., Sperlich, M. A., Ronis, D. L., & Liberzon, I. (2009). Prevalence, trauma history, and risk for posttraumatic stress disorder among nulliparous women in maternity care. *Obstetrics & Gynecology, 114*(4), 839–847.

Setse, R., Grogan, R., Pham, L., Cooper, L. A., Strobino, D., Powe, N. R., & Nicholson, W. (2009). Longitudinal study of depressive symptoms and health-related quality of life during pregnancy and after delivery: The Health Status in Pregnancy (HIP) study. *Maternal Child Health Journal, 13*, 577–587.

Sexton, M. B., Davis, M. T., Menke, R., Raggio, G. A., & Muzik, M. (2017). Mother-child interactions at six months postpartum are not predicted by maternal histories of abuse and neglect or maltreatment type. *Psychological Trauma, 9*(5), 622–626. https://doi.org/http://dx.doi.org/10.1037/tra0000272

Shah, S., & Lonegan, B. (2017). Frequency of postpartum depression and its association with breastfeeding: A cross-sectional survey at immunization clinics in Islamabad, Pakistan. *Journal of the Pakistan Medical Association, 67*, 1151.

Sharma, V., Doobay, M., & Baczynski, C. (2017). Bipolar postpartum depression: An update and recommendations. *Journal of Affective Disorders, 219*, 105–111. https://doi.org/http://dx.doi.org/10.1016/j.jad.2017.05.014

Shaw, J. G., Asch, S. M., Kimerling, R., Frayne, S. M., Shaw, K. A., & Phibbs, C. S. (2014). Posttraumatic stress disorder and risk of spontaneous preterm birth. *Obstetrics & Gynecology, 124*(6), 1111–1119.

Shaw, R. J., Bernard, R. S., DeBlois, T., Ikuta, L. M., Ginzburg, K., & Koopman, C. (2009). The relationship between acute stress disorder and posttraumatic stress disorder in the neonatal intensive care unit. *Psychosomatics, 50*, 131–137.

Shaw, R. J., Deblois, T., Ikuta, L., Ginzburg, K., Fleisher, B., & Koopman, C. (2006). Acute stress disorder among parents of infants in the neonatal intensive care nursery. *Psychosomatics, 47*(3), 206–212. https://doi.org/47/3/206 [pii] 10.1176/appi.psy.47.3.206

Shields, B. (2005). *Down came the rain: My journey through postpartum depression*. Hyperion.

Shirazi, Z. H., Ghasemloo, H., Razavinejad, S. M., Sharifi, N., & Bagheri, S. (2022). The effect of training the fathers to support their wives on stress and self-efficacy in mothers of premature newborns hospitalized in NICU: A quasi-experimental study. *BMC Pregnancy and Childbirth, 22*, 102. https://doi.org/https://doi.org/10.1186/s12884-022-04413-8

Shitu, S., Geda, B., & Dheresa, M. (2019). Postpartum depression and associated factors among mothers who gave birth in the last twelve months in Ankesha District, Awi zone, North West Ethiopia. *BMC Pregnancy and Childbirth, 19*, 435. https://doi.org/https://doi.org/10.1186/s12884-019-2594-y

Silva, C. S., Lima, M. C., Sequeira-de-Andrade, L. A. S., Oliveira, J. S., Monteiro, J. S., Lima, N. M. S., Santos, R. M. A. B., & Lira, P. I. C. (2017). Association between postpartum depression and the practice of exclusive breastfeeding in the first three months of life. *Jornal de Pediatria, 93*(4), 356–364. https://doi.org/http://dx.doi.org/10.1016/j.jped.2016.08.005

Silva, R. S., Azevedo, R., Jr., Sampaio, V. S., Oliveira, K., & Fronza, M. (2021). Postpartum depression: A case-control study. *Journal of Maternal-Fetal & Neonatal Medicine, 34*(17), 2801–2806. https://doi.org/https://doi.org/10.1080/14767058.2019.1671335

Silverman, M. E., & Loudon, H. (2010). Antenatal reports of pre-pregnancy abuse is associated with symptoms of depression in the postpartum period. *Archives of Women's Mental Health, 13*, 411–415.

Simkin, P. (1991). Just another day in a woman's life? Women's long-term perceptions of their first birth experience. Part I. *Birth, 18*(4), 203–210.

Simkin, P. (1992). Just another day in a woman's life? Part II: Nature and consistency of women's long-term memories of their first birth experiences. *Birth, 19*(2), 64–81.

Simpson, M., & Catling, C. (2016). Understanding psychological traumatic birth: A literature review. *Women & Birth, 29*, 203–207.

Sinha, B., Sommerfelt, H., Ashom, P., Mazumder, S., Taneja, S., More, D., & Bahl, R. (2021). Effect of community-initiated kangaroo mother care on postpartum depressive symptoms and stress among mothers of low birthweight infants: A randomized clinical trial. *JAMA Network Open, 4*(4). https://doi.org/10.1001/jamanetworkopen.2021.6040

Skodova, Z., Kelcikova, S., Maskalova, E., & Mazuchova, L. (2022). Infant sleep and temperament characteristics in association with maternal postpartum depression. *Midwifery, 105*, 103232. https://doi.org/https://doi.org/10.1016/j.midw.2021.103232

Slade, P. (2006). Towards a conceptual framework for understanding post-traumatic stress symptoms following childbirth and implications for further research. *Journal of Psychosomatic Obstetrics & Gynecology, 27*(2), 99–105.

Slomian, J., Honvo, G., Emonts, P., Reginster, J.-Y., & Bruyere, O. (2019). Consequences of maternal postpartum depression: A systematic review of maternal and infant outcomes. *Women's Health*, *15*, 1–55. https://doi.org/https://doi.org/10.1177/1745506519844044

Slopen, N., Loucks, E. B., Appleton, A. A., Kawachi, I., Kubzansky, L. D., Non, A. L., Buka, S. L., & Gilman, S. E. (2015). Early origins of inflammation: An examination of prenatal and childhood social adversity in a prospective cohort study. *Psychoneuroendocrinology*, *51*, 403–413.

Smuts, C. M., Huang, M., Mundy, D., Plasse, T., Major, S., & Carlson, S. E. (2003). A randomized trial of docosahexaenoic acid supplementation during the third trimester of pregnancy. *Obstetrics & Gynecology*, *101*, 469–479.

Sockol, L. E., Battle, C. L., Howard, M., & Davis, T. (2014). Correlates of impaired mother-infant bonding in a partial hospital program for perinatal women. *Archives of Women's Mental Health*, *17*, 465–469.

Soderquist, I., Wijma, B., Thorbert, G., & Wijma, K. (2009). Risk factors in pregnancy for posttraumatic stress and depression after childbirth. *British Journal of Obstetrics & Gynecology*, *116*, 672–680.

Sorbo, M. F., Lukasse, M., Brantsaeter, A. L., & Grimstad, H. (2015). Past and recent abuse is associated with early cessation of breast feeding: Results from a large prospective cohort in Norway. *BMJ Open*, *5*(12), 009240.

Speisman, B. B., Storch, E. A., & Abramowitz, J. S. (2011). Postpartum obsessive-compulsive disorder. *Journal of Obstetric, Gynecologic, and Neonatal Nursing*, *40*, 680–690.

Spoormaker, V. I., & Montgomery, P. (2008). Disturbed sleep in post traumatic stress disorder: Secondary symptom or core feature? *Sleep Medicine Reviews*, *12*, 169–184.

Srimoragot, M., Hershberger, P. E., Park, C., Hernandez, T. L., & Balserak, B. I. (2022). Infant feeding type and maternal sleep during the postpartum period: A systematic review and meta-analysis. *Journal of Sleep Research*. https://doi.org/https://doi.org/10.1111/jsr.13625

Stagnaro-Green, A. (2012). Approach to the patient with postpartum thyroiditis. *Journal of Clinical Endocrinology & Metabolism*, *97*, 334–342.

Staneva, A., Bogossian, F., Pritchard, M., & Wittkowski, A. (2015). The effects of maternal depression, anxiety, and perceived stress during pregnancy on preterm birth: A systematic review. *Women & Birth*, *28*(3), 179–193. https://doi.org/10.1016/j.wombi.2015.02.003

Starcevic, V., Eslick, G. D., Viswasam, K., & Berle, D. (2020). Symptoms of obsessive-compulsive disorder during pregnancy and the postpartum period: A systematic review and meta-analysis. *Psychiatric Quarterly*, *91*(4). https://doi.org/10.1007/s11126-020-09769-8

Stepowicz, A., Wencka, B., Bienkiewicz, J., Horzelski, W., & Grzesiak, M. (2020). Stress and anxiety levels in pregnant and postpartum women during the COVID-19 pandemic. *International Journal of Environmental Research and Public Health*, *17*, 9450. https://doi.org/10.3390/ijerph17249450

Stern, G., & Kruckman, L. (1983). Multi-disciplinary perspectives on postpartum depression: An anthropological critique. *Social Science & Medicine*, *17*, 1027–1041.

Stewart, R. C., Umar, E., Tomenson, B., & Creed, F. (2014). A cross-section study of antenatal depression and associated factors in Malawi. *Archives of Women's Mental Health*, *17*, 145–154. https://doi.org/10.1007/s00737-013-0387-2

Stramrood, C. A., Paarlberg, K. M., Velt, E. M. H. I. T., Berger, L. W. A. R., Vingerhoets, A. J. J. M., Schultz, W. C. M. W., & Van Pampus, M. G. (2011). Posttraumatic stress following childbirth in homelike- and hospital settings. *Journal of Psychosomatic Obstetrics & Gynecology*, *32*(2), 88–97.

Strathearn, L., Mamun, A. A., Najman, J. M., & O'Callaghan, M. J. (2009). Does breastfeeding protect against substantiated child abuse and neglect? A 15-year cohort study. *Pediatrics*, *123*(2), 483–493. https://doi.org/123/2/483 [pii] 10.1542/peds.2007-3546

Suarez-Rico, B. V., Estrada-Gutierrez, G., Sanchez-Martinez, M., Perichart-Perera, O., Rodriguez-Hernandez, C., Gonzalez-Leyva, C., Osorio-Valencia, E., Cardona-Perez, A., Helguera-Repetto,

A. C., Espino y Sosa, S., & Solis-Paredes, M. (2021). Prevalence of depression, anxiety, and perceived stress in postpartum Mexican women during the COVID-19 lockdown. *International Journal of Environmental Research and Public Health, 18,* 4627. https://doi.org/https://doi.org/10.3390/ijerph18094627

Sumner, L. A., Wong, L., Schetter, C. D., Myers, H. F., & Rodriguez, M. (2012). Predictors of posttraumatic stress disorder symptoms among low-income Latinas during pregnancy and postpartum. *Psychological Trauma, 4*(2), 196–203.

Szeto, A., Sun-Suslow, N., Mendez, A. J., Hernandez, R. I., Wagner, K., & McCabe, P. M. (2017). Regulation of the macrophage oxytocin receptor response to inflammation. *American Journal of Physiology, Endocrinology, and Metabolism, 312*(3), E183–E189. https://doi.org/10.1152/ajpendo.00346.2016

Taveras, E. M., Rifas-Shiman, S. L., Rich-Edwards, J. W., & Mantzoros, C. S. (2011). Maternal short sleep duration associated with increased levels of inflammatory markers at 3 years postpartum. *Metabolism, 60*(7), 982–986.

Tavoli, Z., Tavoli, A., Amirpour, R., Hosseini, R., & Montazeri, A. (2016). Quality of life in women who were exposed to domestic violence during pregnancy. *BMC Pregnancy and Childbirth, 16,* 19. https://doi.org/10.1186/s12884-016-0810-6

Tebeka, S., Le Strat, Y., Mandelbrot, I., Benachi, A., Dommergues, M., Kayem, G., Lepercq, J., Luton, D., Ville, Y., Ramoz, N., Mulbert, J., Dubertret, C., & IGEDEPP Groups. (2021). Early- and late-onset postpartum depression exhibit distinct associated factors: The IGEDEPP prospective cohort study. *British Journal of Obstetrics & Gynaecology, 128,* 1683–1693. https://doi.org/10.1111/1471-0528.16688

Tees, M. T., Harville, E. W., Xiong, X., Buekens, P., Pridjian, G., & Elkind-Hirsch, K. (2010). Hurricane Katrina-related maternal stress, maternal mental health, and early infant temperament. *Maternal & Child Health Journal, 14*(4), 511–518.

Tham, V., Ryding, E. L., & Christensson, K. (2010). Experience of support among mothers with and without post-traumatic symptoms following emergency caesarean section. *Sexual & Reproductive Healthcare, 1,* 175–190.

Thul, T. A., Corwin, E. J., Carlson, N. S., Brennan, P. A., & Young, L. J. (2020). Oxytocin and postpartum depression: A systematic review. *Psychoneuroendocrinology, 120.* https://doi.org/https://doi.org/10.1016/j.psyneuen.2020.104793

Tietz, A., Zietlow, A.-L., & Reck, C. (2014). Maternal bonding in mothers with postpartum anxiety disorder: The crucial role of subclinical depressive symptoms and maternal avoidance behaviour. *Archives of Women's Mental Health, 17,* 433–442.

Tobback, E., Behaeghel, K., Hanoulle, I., Delesie, L., Loccufier, A., van Holsbeeck, A., & Vogelaers, D. (2017). Comparison of subjective sleep and fatigue in breast- and bottle-feeding mothers. *Midwifery, 47,* 22–27. https://doi.org/http://dx.doi.org/10.1016/j.midw.2017.01.009

Torchalla, I., Linden, I. A., Strehlau, V., Neilson, E. K., & Krausz, M. (2015). "Like a lot happened with my whole childhood": Violence, trauma, and addiction in pregnant and postpartum women from Vancouver's Downtown Eastside. *Harm Reduction Journal, 12*(1). www.harmreductionjournal.com/content/12/1/1

Torkan, B., Parsay, S., Lamyian, M., Kazemnejad, A., & Montazeri, A. (2009). Postnatal quality of life in women after normal vaginal delivery vs caesarean section. *BMC Pregnancy and Childbirth, 9*(4). https://doi.org/10.1186/1471-2393-9-4

Toru, T., Chemir, F., & Anand, S. (2018). Magnitude of postpartum depression and associated factors among women in Mizan Aman town, Bench Maji zone, Southwest Ethiopia. *BMC Pregnancy and Childbirth, 18,* 442. https://doi.org/https://doi.org/10.1186/s12884-018-2072-y

Tran, L. M., Nguyen, P. H., Naved, R. T., & Menon, P. (2020). Intimate partner violence is associated with poorer mental health and breastfeeding practices in Bangladesh. *Health Policy & Planning, 35*(Suppl. 1), i19–i29. https://doi.org/10.1093/heapol/czaa106

Turkcapar, A. F., Kadioglu, N., Aslan, E., Tunc, S., Zayifoglu, M., & Mollamahmutoglu, L. (2015). Sociodemographic and clinical feature of postpartum depression among Turkish women: A prospective study. *BMC Pregnancy and Childbirth*, *15*, 108. 10.1186/s12884-015-0532-1

Turkmen, H., Dilcen, H. Y., & Akin, B. (2020). The effect of labor comfort on traumatic childbirth perception, posttraumatic stress disorder, and breastfeeding. *Breastfeeding Medicine*, *15*(12), 779–788. https://doi.org/10.1089/bfm.2020.0138

Uchino, B. N., Trettevik, R., Kent de Grey, R. G., Cronan, S., Hogan, J., & Baucom, B. R. W. (2018). Social support, social integration, and inflammatory cytokines: A meta-analysis. *Health Psychology*, *37*(5), 462–471.

Uvnas-Moberg, K. (2013). *The hormone of closeness: The role of oxytocin in relationships*. Pinter & Martin.

Uvnas-Moberg, K. (2015). *Oxytocin: The biological guide to motherhood*. Praeclarus Press.

Uvnas-Moberg, K., Ekstrom-Bergstrom, A., Buckley, S., Massarotti, C., Pajalic, Z., Luegmair, K., Kotiowska, A., Lengier, L., Olza, I., Grylka-Baeschlin, S., Leahy-Warren, P., Hadjigeorgiu, E., Valliarmea, S., & Dencker, A. (2020). Maternal plasma levels of oxytocin during breastfeeding. *PLoS One*, *15*(8), e0235806. https://doi.org/10.1371/journal.pone.0235806

Valentine, J. M., Rodriguez, M. A., Lapeyrouse, L. M., & Zhang, M. (2011). Recent intimate partner violence as a prenatal predictor of maternal depression in the first year postpartum among Latinas. *Archives of Women's Mental Health*, *14*, 135–143.

Valla, L., Helseth, S., Smastuen, M. C., Misvaer, N., & Andenaes, R. (2022). Factors associated with maternal overall quality of life at six months postpartum: A cross-sectional study from the Norwegian mother, father, and child cohort study. *BMC Pregnancy and Childbirth*, *22*, 4. https://doi.org/https://doi.org/10.1186/s12884-021-04303-5

van Bussel, J. C. H., Spitz, B., & Demyttenaere, K. (2009). Depressives symptomatology in pregnant and postpartum women: An exploratory study of the role of maternal antenatal orientations. *Archives of Women's Mental Health*, *12*, 155–163.

Vanderbilt, D., Bushley, T., Young, R., & Frank, D. A. (2009). Acute posttraumatic stress symptoms among urban mothers with newborns in the neonatal intensive care unit: A preliminary study. *Journal of Developmental & Behavioral Pediatrics*, *30*, 50–56.

van der Zee-van den Berg, A. I., Boere-Boonekamp, M. M., Groothuis-Oudshoorn, M., & Reijneveld, S. A. (2021). Postpartum depression and anxiety: A community-based study on risk factors before, during, and after pregnancy. *Journal of Affective Disorders*, *286*, 158–165. https://doi.org/https://doi.org/10.1016/j.jad.2021.02.062

Varin, M., Palladino, E., Orpana, H. M., Wong, S. L., Gheorghe, M., Lary, T., & Baker, M. M. (2020). Prevalence of positive mental health and associated factors among postpartum women in Canada: Findings from a national cross-sectional survey. *Maternal & Child Health Journal*, *24*, 759–767. https://doi.org/http://dx.doi.org/10.1016/j.midw.2017.01.009

Vericker, T. C. (2015). *Maternal depression associated with less healthy dietary behaviors in young children*. www.urban.org

Verreault, N., Da Costa, D., Marchand, A., Ireland, K., Banack, H., Dritsa, M., & Khalife, S. (2012). PTSD following childbirth: A prospective study of incidence and risk factors in Canadian women. *Journal of Psychosomatic Research*, *73*, 257–263.

Wakeel, F., Wisk, L. E., Gee, R., Chao, S. M., & Witt, W. P. (2013). The balance between and personal capital during pregnancy and the relationship with adverse obstetric outcomes: Findings from the 2007 Los Angeles Mommy and Baby (LAMB) study. *Archives of Women's Mental Health*, *16*, 435–451.

Walker, A. L., de Rooij, S. R., Dimitrova, M. V., Witteveen, A. B., Verhoeven, C. J., de Jonge, A., Vridkotte, T. G. M., & Henrichs, J. (2021). Psychosocial and peripartum determinants of postpartum depression: Findings from a prospective population-based cohort. The ABCD study. *Comprehensive Psychiatry*, *108*. https://doi.org/https://doi.org/10.1016/j.comppsych.2021.152239

Walker, E. R., McGee, R. E., & Druss, B. G. (2015). Mortality in mental disorders and global disease burden implications: A systematic review and meta-analysis. *JAMA Psychiatry*, 72, 334–341. https://doi.org/10.1001/jamapsychiatry.2014.2502

Walmer, R., Huynh, J., Wenger, J., Ankers, E., Mantha, A. B., Ecker, J., & Thadhani, R. (2015). Mental health disorders subsequent to gestational diabetes mellitus differ by race/ethnicity. *Depression & Anxiety*, 32, 774–782.

Walters, C. N., Rakotomanana, H., Komakech, J. J., & Stoecker, B. J. (2021). Maternal experience of intimate partner violence is associated with suboptimal breastfeeding practices in Malawi, Tanzania, and Zambia: Insights from a DHS analysis. *International Breastfeeding Journal*, 16(1), 20. https://doi.org/10.1186/s13006-021-00365-5

Wang, D. X., Li, Y.-L., Qiu, D., & Xiao, S.-Y. (2021). Factors influencing paternal postpartum depression: A systematic review and meta-analysis. *Journal of Affective Disorders*, 293, 51–63. https://doi.org/https://doi.org/10.1016/j.jad.2021.05.088

Watkins, S., Meltzer-Brody, S., Zolnoun, D., & Stuebe, A. M. (2011). Early breastfeeding experiences and postpartum depression *Obstetrics & Gynecology*, 118(2), 214–221.

Webber, S. (1992). Supporting the postpartum family. *The Doula*, 23, 16–17.

Webber, S. (2012). *The gentle art of newborn family care*. Praeclarus Press.

Webster, J., Linnane, J. W. J., Dibley, L. M., & Pritchard, M. (2000). Improving antenatal recognition of women at risk for postnatal depression. *Australia and New Zealand Journal of Obstetrics and Gynaecology*, 40, 409–412.

Weisman, O., Granat, A., Gilboa-Schechtman, E., Singer, M., Gordon, I., Azulay, H., Kuint, J., & Feldman, R. (2010). The experience of labor, maternal perception of the infant, and the mother's postpartum mood in a low-risk community cohort. *Archives of Women's Mental Health*, 13, 505–513.

Weissman, M. M., Pilowsky, D. J., Wickramaratne, P. J., Talati, A., Wisniewski, S. R., Fava, M., Hughes, C. W., Garber, J., Malloy, E., King, C. A., & Cerda, G. (2006). Remissions in maternal depression and child psychopathology. *JAMA*, 295(12), 1389–1398.

Williams, K. E., & Koleva, H. (2018). Identification and treatment of peripartum anxiety disorders. *Obstetric & Gynecology Clinics*, 45(3), 469–481.

Wilson, N., Lee, J. J., & Bei, B. (2019). Postpartum fatigue and depression: A systematic review and meta-analysis. *Journal of Affective Disorders*, 246, 224–233.

Wolke, D., Rizzo, P., & Woods, S. (2002). Persistent infant crying and hyperactivity problems in middle childhood. *Pediatrics*, 109, 1054–1060.

Woolhouse, H., Brown, S., Krastev, A., Perlen, S., & Gunn, J. (2009). Seeking help for anxiety and depression after childbirth: Results of the maternal health study. *Archives of Disease of Childhood*, 12, 75–83.

Woolhouse, H., Gartland, D., Mensah, F., & Brown, S. J. (2015). Maternal depression from early pregnancy to 4 years postpartum in a prospective pregnancy cohort study: Implications for primary health care. *British Journal of Obstetrics & Gynecology*, 122, 312–321. https://doi.org/10.1111/1471-0528.12839

Woolhouse, H., James, J., Gartland, D., McDonald, E., & Brown, S. J. (2016). Maternal depressive symptoms at three months postpartum and breastfeeding rates at six months postpartum: Implications for primary care in a prospective cohort study of primiparous women in Australia. *Women & Birth*, 29(4), 381–387. https://doi.org/10.1016/j.wombi.2016.05.008

World Health Organization. (2014). *The prevention and elimination of disrespect and abuse during facility-based childbirth*. http://apps.who.int/iris/bitstream/10665/134588/1/WHO_RHR_14.23_eng.pdf?ua=1&ua=1

Worthen, R. J., & Beurel, E. (2022). Inflammatory and neurodegenerative pathophysiology implicated in postpartum depression. *Neurobiology of Disease*, 165, 1056–1046. https://doi.org/https://doi.org/10.1016/j.nbd.2022.105646

Xiong, P. T., Poehlmann, J., Stowe, Z., & Antony, K. M. (2021). Anxiety, depression, and pain in the perinatal period: A review for obstetric care providers. *Obstetrical & Gynecological Survey*, 76(11), 692–713. https://doi.org/10.1097/OGX.0000000000000958

Xiong, X., Harville, E. W., Mattison, D. R., Elkind-Hirsch, K., Pridjian, G., & Buekens, P. (2010). Hurricane Katrina experience and the risk of post-traumatic stress disorder and depression among pregnant women. *American Journal of Disaster Medicine*, 5(3), 181–187.

Yakupova, V., Suarez, A., & Kharchenko, A. (2022). Birth experience, postpartum PTSD, and depression before and during the pandemic of COVID-19 in Russia. *International Journal of Environmental Research and Public Health*, 19. https://doi.org/https://doi.org/10.3390/ijerph19010335

Yatham, L. N., Kennedy, S. H., Schaffer, A., Parikh, S. V., Beaulieu, S., O'Donovan, C., MacQueen, G., McIntyre, R. S., Sharma, V., Ravindran, A., & Young, L. T. (2009). Canadian Network for Mood and Anxiety Treatments (CANMAT) and International Society for Bipolar Disorders (ISBD) collaborative update of CANMAT guidelines for the management of patients with bipolar disorder: Update 2009. *Bipolar Disorders*, 11, 225–255.

Yim, I. S., Glynn, L. M., Schetter, C. D., Hobel, C. J., Chicz-DeMet, A., & Sandman, C. A. (2009). Risk of postpartum depressive symptoms with elevated corticotropin-releasing hormone in human pregnancy. *Archives General Psychiatry*, 66(2), 162–169.

Yonkers, K. A., Smith, M. V., Forray, A., Epperson, C. N., Costello, D., Lin, H., & Belanger, K. (2014). Pregnant women with posttraumatic stress disorder and risk of preterm birth. *JAMA Psychiatry*, 71(8), 897–904.

Yusuff, A. S. M., Tang, L., Binns, C. W., & Lee, A. H. (2016). Breastfeeding and postnatal depression: A prospective cohort study in Sabah, Malaysia. *Journal of Human Lactation*, 32(2), 277–281.

Zafar, S., Jean-Baptiste, R., Rahman, A., Neilson, J. P., & van den Broek, N. (2015). Non-life threatening maternal morbidity: Cross-sectional surveys from Malawi and Pakistan. *PLoS One*, 10. https://doi.org/10260.1371/journal.pone.0138026

Index

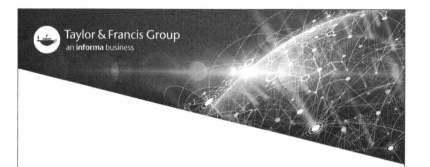

Printed in the United States
by Baker & Taylor Publisher Services